Curbside Consultation in Refractive and Lens-Based Surgery

49 Clinical Questions

T0312866

Curbside Consultation in Ophthalmology
SERIES

SERIES EDITOR, DAVID F. CHANG, MD

Curbside Consultation in Refractive and Lens-Based Surgery

49 Clinical Questions

Editors

Bonnie An Henderson, MD
Clinical Professor of Ophthalmology
Tufts University School of Medicine
Ophthalmic Consultants of Boston
Boston, Massachusetts

Sonia H. Yoo, MD
Professor of Ophthalmology
Bascom Palmer Eye Institute
University of Miami
Miller School of Medicine
Miami, Florida

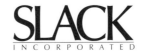

SLACK
INCORPORATED

www.Healio.com/books

ISBN: 978-1-61711-083-2

SLACK Incorporated uses a review process to evaluate submitted material. Prior to publication, educators or clinicians provide important feedback on the content that we publish. We welcome feedback on this work.

Published by: SLACK Incorporated
                         6900 Grove Road
                         Thorofare, NJ 08086 USA
                         Telephone: 856-848-1000
                         Fax: 856-848-6091
                         www.Healio.com/books

Contact SLACK Incorporated for more information about other books in this field or about the availability of our books from distributors outside the United States.

Library of Congress Cataloging-in-Publication Data

Curbside consultation in refractive and lens-based surgery : 49 clinical questions / editors, Bonnie An Henderson, Sonia H. Yoo.
    p. ; cm. -- (Curbside consultation in ophthalmology series)
  Includes bibliographical references and index.
  ISBN 978-1-61711-083-2 (alk. paper)
  I. Henderson, Bonnie An, editor. II. Yoo, Sonia H., 1966- , editor. III. Series: Curbside consultation in ophthalmology series.
  [DNLM: 1. Refractive Surgical Procedures--methods. WW 340]
  RE925
  617.7'55--dc23
                      2014026110

Dedication

To our colleagues for always being open to a curbside consultation.
To our challengers for giving us the motivation to persevere.
To our loved ones for giving us the support to continue every day.

Contents

Acknowledgments

This series of *Curbside Consultation* books is the brainchild of Dr. David Chang. Like everything he does, David thoughtfully crafted a collection of books that focus on the most common, but crucial topics in each of the specialties. Without David's vision, this useful reference would never have materialized.

We would like to thank all the authors for contributing their sage advice. We realize that everyone is incredibly busy and writing a book chapter is a very generous donation of time. Writing a book chapter is truly a labor of love with no remuneration, except a grateful handshake and a free copy of the book. We also thank their families for allowing them to take on this additional project which undoubtedly took away from their personal time.

Finally, we would like to thank John Bond at SLACK along with his team, Tony Schiavo, Jean-Marc Yee, Michelle Gatt, Catherine Girone, and April Billick. Their expert guidance, input, and gentle prodding was the secret sauce for the successful completion of this book.

About the Editors

Bonnie An Henderson, MD is a partner at Ophthalmic Consultants of Boston and a Clinical Professor at Tufts University School of Medicine. Dr. Henderson completed her ophthalmology residency at Harvard Medical School, Massachusetts Eye and Ear Infirmary. She graduated from Dartmouth College and from Dartmouth Medical School with high honors. Dr. Henderson specializes in refractive cataract surgery and complex anterior segment surgery. She has authored over 100 articles, papers, book chapters, and abstracts, written/edited 4 textbooks, and has delivered over 250 invited lectures worldwide. Dr. Henderson is the Associate Editor for the *Journal of Refractive Surgery* and Associate Editor for *Eyeworld* for the American Society of Cataract and Refractive Surgery. She serves on the editorial advisory board of *Eyenet Magazine* of the American Academy of Ophthalmology, and serves on the editorial boards of 3 other journals. She serves on a number of committees for the American Academy of Ophthalmology and the American Society of Cataract and Refractive Society. She is a reviewer for eight ophthalmic journals.

Dr. Henderson has been awarded an Achievement Award and Secretariat Award by the American Academy of Ophthalmology, and "Best of" awards from the American Society of Cataract and Refractive Surgery for her research and films. She serves on the Executive Committee and is the President-Elect of the American Society of Cataract and Refractive Surgery for 2017. She serves on the Executive Board of the Massachusetts Society of Eye Physicians and Surgeons, the Executive Board of Women In Ophthalmology, and has served on the Physician Board of Directors at the Massachusetts Eye and Ear Infirmary. She also serves on the Board of Overseers at the Geisel School of Medicine at Dartmouth.

Sonia H. Yoo, MD is a Professor of Ophthalmology with a joint appointment in Biomedical Engineering and Associate Medical Director at Bascom Palmer Eye Institute, University of Miami, Miller School of Medicine. Dr. Yoo received her BA at Stanford University and MD at Case Western Reserve University. She completed residency and fellowship at Massachusetts Eye and Ear Infirmary, Harvard Medical School in 1998.

Her areas of clinical practice are cornea, cataract, and refractive surgery. Her areas of research interest are in laser applications in cornea, cataract, and refractive surgery and restoring accommodation. She has authored over 100 book chapters and peer-reviewed journal articles and has been the principle investigator in numerous drug and device trials. Dr. Yoo served as the cornea fellowship director at Bascom Palmer Eye Institute from 2000-2013.

Dr. Yoo is the 2014 program chair of the Refractive Surgery subspecialty day program of the American Academy of Ophthalmology and serves on the Academy's Practicing Ophthalmologists Curriculum Refractive Management/Intervention Panel for refractive surgery. She is a board member of the American Society of Cataract and Refractive Surgery and is on the board of directors for the Cornea Society. She is a reviewer for numerous peer-reviewed journals. Additionally, she serves on the editorial board of the *Cornea Society*, the *Journal of Refractive Surgery*, the *Journal of Cataract and Refractive Surgery*, and *Ophthalmic Surgery, Lasers and Imaging*.

Contributing Authors

Alessandro Abbouda, MD (Chapter 20)
Clinical Research Fellow in Vissum Corporation
Alicante, Spain
Resident in University of Rome "Sapienza"
Rome, Italy
Department of Ophthalmology
Policlinico Umberto I of Rome
Rome, Italy

Natalie Afshari, MD, FACS (Chapter 38)
Stuart I Brown MD Chair in Ophthalmology
  in Memory of Donald P. Shiley
Professor of Ophthalmology
Chief of Cornea & Refractive Surgery
Shiley Eye Center
University of California
San Diego, California

Jorge L. Alió, MD, PhD (Chapter 20)
Medical Director
VISSUM Corporation
Alicante, Spain
Professor and Chairman of Ophthalmology
Miguel Hernández University
Alicante, Spain

Zaina Al-Mohtaseb (Chapter 30)
Instructor of Ophthalmology
Cullen Eye Institute
Baylor College of Medicine
Houston, Texas

Renato Ambrósio Jr, MD, PhD (Chapter 22)
Associate Professor of Ophthalmology
Federal University of São Paulo
Founder and Scientific Director of the
  Rio de Janeiro Corneal Tomography and
  Biomechanics Study Group
São Paulo, Brazil

Samuel Arba Mosquera, PhD, MSc (Chapter 9)
Optical/Visual Researcher
R&D Department
SCHWIND Eye-Tech-Solutions GmbH &
  Co. KG
Kleinostheim, Germany

John P. Berdahl, MD (Chapter 33)
Vance Thompson Vision
Sioux Falls, South Dakota

Hiroko Bissen-Miyajima, MD, PhD (Chapter 46)
Professor and Department Chair
Tokyo Dental College Suidobashi Hospital
Tokyo, Japan

Ofelia Brugnoli de Pagano, MD (Chapter 2)
Associate Professor
Ophthalmology Department
Universidad Nacional de Cuyo
Mendoza, Argentina
Head of Strabismus
Department at the Hospital Central de
  Mendoza
Mendoza, Argentina
Strabismus and Refractive Surgery Specialist
Centrovision Mendoza Eye Clinic
Mendoza, Argentina

Florence Cabot, MD (Chapter 21)
Bascom Palmer Eye Institute
University of Miami
Miller School of Medicine
Miami, Florida

Francesco Carones, MD (Chapter 27)
Medical Director and CEO
Carones Ophthalmology Center
Milan, Italy

Jessica B. Ciralsky, MD (Chapter 25)
Assistant Professor of Ophthalmology
Weill Cornell Medical College
New York, New York

Rosane de Oliveira Corrêa, MD (Chapter 22)
Assistant Ophthalmologist
Instituto de Olhos Renato Ambrósio
Ophthalmologist of the Rio de Janeiro Corneal
  Tomography and Biomechanics Study Group
Rio de Janeiro, Brazil

William W. Culbertson, MD (Chapter 17)
Professor of Ophthalmology
Bascom Palmer Eye Institute
University of Miami
Miller School of Medicine
Miami, Florida

Yassine J. Daoud, MD (Chapter 1)
Assistant Professor of Ophthalmology
Cornea, Cataract, and Refractive Surgery
  Services
Wilmer Eye Institute
Johns Hopkins Medical Institutions
Baltimore, Maryland

*Mahshad Darvish-Zargar, MD CM, MBA,
  FRCSC (Chapter 28)*
McGill University
Department of Ophthalmology
Jewish General Hospital
Montreal, Quebec

Elizabeth A. Davis, MD, FACS (Chapter 24)
Partner, Minnesota Eye Consultants
Adjunct Clinical Assistant Professor
University of Minnesota
Minneapolis, Minnesota

*Uday Devgan, MD, FACS, FRCS(Glasg)
  (Chapter 35)*
Private Practice
Devgan Eye Surgery
Los Angeles, California
Specialty Surgical Center
Beverly Hills, California
Chief of Ophthalmology
Olive View UCLA
Medical Center Associate
Clinical Professor of Ophthalmology
Jules Stein Eye Institute
UCLA School of Medicine
Los Angeles, California

Deepinder K. Dhaliwal, MD, LAc (Chapter 31)
Associate Professor of Ophthalmology
University of Pittsburgh School of Medicine
Director
Cornea Service Director
Refractive Surgery Service Founder and
  Director
Center for Integrative Eye Care
Director, Cornea and Refractive Surgery
  Fellowship Program Medical Director,
  UPMC Laser Vision/Aesthetic Center
University of Pittsburgh Medical Center
Pittsburgh, Pennsylvania

Vasilios F. Diakonis, MD, PhD (Chapters 13, 14)
Bascom Palmer Eye Institute
Miller School of Medicine
University of Miami
Miami, Florida

Eric D. Donnenfeld, MD (Chapter 18)
Clinical Professor of Ophthalmology
New York University Medical Center
New York, New York

Jason N. Edmonds, MD (Chapter 16)
Clinical Instructor
Department of Ophthalmology and Visual
  Sciences
John A. Moran Eye Center
University of Utah, School of Medicine
Salt Lake City, Utah

Damien Gatinel, MD (Chapter 3, 7)
Assistant Professor of Ophthalmology
Head of Cataract, Anterior Segment and
  Refractive Surgery Department
Rothschild Foundation
Paris, France

Ramon Coral Ghanem, MD, PhD (Chapter 5)
Cornea and Refractive Surgery Department
Sadalla Amin Ghanem Eye Hospital
Joinville/SC, Brazil

Vinícius Coral Ghanem, MD, PhD (Chapter 5)
Cornea and Refractive Surgery Department
Sadalla Amin Ghanem Eye Hospital
Joinville/SC, Brazil

Preeya K. Gupta, MD (Chapter 26)
Assistant Professor of Ophthalmology
Cornea & Refractive Surgery
Clinical Director Duke Eye Center at Page
  Road
Duke University Eye Center
Durham, North Carolina

David R. Hardten, MD (Chapter 37)
Director of Clinical Research
Minnesota Eye Consultants
Minneapolis, Minnesota
Adjunct Associate Professor of Ophthalmology
University of Minnesota
Minneapolis, Minnesota

Lingmin He, MD, MS (Chapter 12)
Byers Eye Institute
Stanford Hospital & Clinics
Palo Alto, California

Richard S. Hoffman, MD (Chapter 49)
Clinical Associate Professor of Ophthalmology
Casey Eye Institute
Oregon Health and Science University
Portland, Oregon

Edward J. Holland, MD (Chapter 28)
Director of Cornea
Cincinnati Eye Institute
Professor of Ophthalmology
University of Cincinnati
Cincinnati, Ohio

Yoshihiko Iida, MD, PhD (Chapter 40)
Assistant Professor
Department of Ophthalmology
Kitasato University School of Medicine
Sagamihara, Japan

A.J. Kanellopoulos, MD (Chapter 8)
Medical Director
Laservision.gr Institute
Athens, Greece
Clinical Professor of Ophthalmology
NYU Medical School
New York, New York

Vardhaman P. Kankariya, MD (Chapters 10, 13, 14)
Bascom Palmer Eye Institute
Miller School of Medicine
University of Miami
Miami, Florida

Sumitra S. Khandelwal, MD (Chapters 24, 37)
Assistant Professor
Cullen Eye Institute
Baylor College of Medicine
Houston, Texas

Wei Boon Khor, MBBS, FRCSEd (Chapter 38)
Consultant
Cornea and External Eye Disease Service
Singapore National Eye Centre
Adjunct Assistant Professor
Duke-NUS Graduate Medical School
Singapore

Jae Yong Kim, MD, PhD (Chapter 41)
Associate Professor
Department of Ophthalmology
University of Ulsan College of Medicine
Asan Medical Center
Seoul, South Korea

Terry Kim, MD (Chapter 44)
Professor of Ophthalmology
Duke University School of Medicine
Director of Fellowship Programs
Cornea and Refractive Surgery Services
Duke University Eye Center
Durham, North Carolina

Michael C. Knorz, MD (Chapter 23)
Professor of Ophthalmology
Medical Faculty
Mannheim of the University of Heidelberg
Mannheim, Germany

Douglas D. Koch, MD (Chapter 30)
Professor and Allen, Law, and Mosbacher
  Chair in Ophthalmology
Cullen Eye Institute
Baylor College of Medicine
Houston, Texas

George A. Kontadakis, MD, MSc (Chapter 11)
Clinical and Research Fellow
Institute of Vision and Optics
University of Crete
Greece

George D. Kymionis, MD, PhD (Chapter 11)
Assistant Professor of Ophthalmology
Medical School
University of Crete
Greece
Vol. Assistant Professor
Bascom Palmer Eye Institute
University of Miami
Miami, Florida

Edward C. Lai, MD (Chapter 25)
Assistant Professor of Ophthalmology
Weill Cornell Medical College
New York, New York

Richard L. Lindstrom, MD (Chapter 37)
Founder and Attending Surgeon
Minnesota Eye Consultants
Adjunct Professor Emeritus
University of Minnesota
Department of Ophthalmology
Visiting Professor
UC Irvine's Gavin Herbert Eye Institute
Irvine, California

Jordon G. Lubahn, MD (Chapter 17)
Bascom Palmer Eye Institute
University of Miami
Miami, Florida

Kim-Binh Mai, MD (Chapter 36)
The University of Texas Medical School at
  Houston and Ruiz
Department of Ophthalmology and Visual
  Science
University of Texas
Houston, Texas

Alex Mammen, MD (Chapter 31)
Clinical Assistant Professor of Ophthalmology
University of Pittsburgh Medical Center
Pittsburgh, Pennsylvania

Edward E. Manche, MD (Chapter 12)
Director of Cornea and Refractive Surgery
Professor of Ophthalmology
Stanford University School of Medicine
Stanford, California

Jay J. Meyer, MD, MPH (Chapter 26)
Clinical Associate
Duke University Eye Center
Durham, North Carolina

Kevin M. Miller, MD (Chapter 32)
Kolokotrones   Professor   of   Clinical
  Ophthalmology
Jules Stein Eye Institute
David Geffen School of Medicine at UCLA
Los Angeles, California

Majid Moshirfar, MD (Chapter 16)
Professor of Ophthalmology
Clinical Instructor
Department of Ophthalmology and Visual
  Sciences
John A. Moran Eye Center
University of Utah, School of Medicine
Salt Lake City, Utah

Afshan Nanji, MD, MPH (Chapter 6)
Instructor
Department of Ophthalmology
Bascom Palmer Eye Institute
Miami, Florida

Louis D. "Skip" Nichamin, MD (Chapter 47)
Private Ophthalmic Surgeon and Consultant
Laurel Eye Clinic
Brookville, Pennsylvania

Rudy M. M. A. Nuijts, MD, PhD (Chapter 29)
Professor in Ophthalmology
University Eye Clinic
Maastricht University Medical Center
Maastricht, Netherlands

Mark Packer, MD, FACS, CPI (Chapter 45)
Clinical Associate Professor
Oregon Health & Science University
Director, Bowie Vision Institute
Bowie, Maryland

Gabriela L. Pagano, MD (Chapter 2)
Cornea and Refractive Surgery Specialist at
  Centrovision Mendoza Eye Clinic
Mendoza, Argentina
Assistant Professor
Ophthalmology Department
Universidad Nacional de Cuyo
Mendoza, Argentina
Former Cornea and Refractive Surgery Fellow
Instituto de Oftalmologia Conde de Valenciana
Mexico City, Mexico

Parag Parekh, MD, MPA (Chapter 47)
Laurel Eye Clinic
Brookville, Pennsylvania

Jay S. Pepose, MD, PhD (Chapter 39)
Founder and Medical Director
Pepose Vision Institute
Professor of Clinical Ophthalmology
Washington University School of Medicine
St. Louis, Missouri

J. Bradley Randleman, MD (Chapter 4)
Professor of Ophthalmology
Director, Cornea, External Disease, &
  Refractive Surgery
Emory University Department of
  Ophthalmology
Atlanta, Georgia
Editor-In-Chief, *Journal of Refractive Surgery*

Peter A. Rapoza, MD, FACS (Chapter 48)
Assistant Clinical Professor
Harvard Medical School
Department of Ophthalmology
Massachusetts Eye and Ear Infirmary
Boston, Massachusetts

Sherman Reeves, MD (Chapter 37)
Partner, Minnesota Eye Consultants
Adjunct Assistant Professor of Ophthalmology
University of Minnesota
Minneapolis, Minnesota

Alain Saad, MD (Chapter 3)
Ophthalmologist
Anterior Segment and Refractive Surgery
  Department
Rothschild Foundation
Paris, France

Matthew J. Schear, DO (Chapter 18)
Department of Ophthalmology
Hofstra North Shore - LIJ
Hofstra University
Hempstead, New York

Kimiya Shimizu, MD, PhD (Chapter 40)
Professor and Chair
Department of Ophthalmology
Kitasato University School of Medicine
Sagamihara, Japan

Walter J. Stark, MD (Chapter 1)
Boone Pickens Professor of Ophthalmology
Director of Stark-Mosher Center for Cataract
  and Corneal Services
Johns Hopkins University School of Medicine
Wilmer Eye Institute
Baltimore, Maryland

Roger F. Steinert, MD (Chapter 42)
Irving H. Leopold Professor
Professor of Biomedical Engineering
Chair of Ophthalmology
Director, Gavin Herbert Eye Institute
University of California
Irvine, California

Richard Tipperman, MD (Chapter 43)
Attending Surgeon
Wills Eye Hospital
Philadelphia, Pennsylvania

William Trattler, MD (Chapter 22)
Director of Cornea
Center For Excellence In Eye Care
Miami, Florida

Pravin Krishna Vaddavalli, MD (Chapter 10)
Cornea Service
Head, Refractive Surgery and Cataract Service
LV Prasad Eye Institute
Hyderabad, India

Bruna V. Ventura, MD, MS (Chapter 30)
Ophthalmologist
Altino Ventura Foundation and HOPE Eye
  Hospital
Recife, Brazil

Laura Vickers, MD (Chapter 44)
Chief Resident
Duke University Eye Center
Durham, North Carolina

Nienke Visser, MD (Chapter 29)
Resident and PhD Student in Ophthalmology
University Eye Clinic
Maastricht University Medical Center
Maastricht, Netherlands

R. Bruce Wallace III, MD, FACS (Chapter 34)
Clinical Professor of Ophthalmology
Tulane Medical School
LSU School of Medicine
New Orleans, Louisiana

Li Wang, MD, PhD (Chapter 30)
Associate Professor of Ophthalmology
Cullen Eye Institute
Baylor College of Medicine
Houston, Texas

Matthew J. Weiss, MD (Chapter 15)
Cornea and Refractive Surgery Fellow: Bascom
  Palmer Eye Institute, University of Miami
  Miller School of Medicine
Miami, Florida

Roberto Zaldivar, MD (Chapter 19)
Scientific Director
Instituto Zaldivar
Mendoza, Argentina

Roger Zaldivar, MD (Chapter 19)
Medical Director
Instituto Zaldivar
Mendoza, Argentina

Preface

The *Curbside Consultation* series continues to be one of the most common resources clinicians turn to when faced with a difficult patient scenario. Bonnie and I have had twenty years of curbside consulting back and forth between us starting from residency and throughout our careers. We have on occasion been known to "phone a friend" when needing advice on a tricky situation. This book on refractive and lens-based surgery is a compilation of real-life clinical scenarios that we have encountered in our practices. We have asked our colleagues, specialists who we would call for advice, to respond to these questions in an informal format, as if talking to a colleague on the phone or by email.

We have divided the book into corneal refractive surgery and lens-based surgery and within each section, have further divided it into preoperative, intraoperative and postoperative questions. The responses from our authors are based upon their personal experience with support from the peer-reviewed literature.

We hope you find the textbook practical and concise. Our goal is to present questions that you may face in your refractive practice and give you answers that may not be readily available in the scientific journals.

Bonnie An Henderson, MD
Sonia H. Yoo, MD

SECTION I

PREOPERATIVE CONSULTATION

MY PATIENT HAS A SYSTEMIC DISEASE.
SHOULD I PERFORM REFRACTIVE SURGERY?

Yassine J. Daoud, MD and Walter J. Stark, MD

Laser refractive surgery (LRS) is a common and popular procedure. As the successful outcomes of LRS are highlighted in the popular culture, patients, including those with underlying systemic diseases, are inquiring about such procedures.

This specific patient population presents a dilemma because the refractive error is accompanied by a systemic disease that may have an ocular or corneal component. Further, the underlying disorder may cause intraoperative or postoperative complications that are not encountered in otherwise healthy patients.

The United States Food and Drug Administration (FDA) established a list of ocular and systemic contraindications to photorefractive keratectomy (PRK) in the mid 1990s; this list included diabetes mellitus (DM), collagen vascular diseases (CVD) such as rheumatoid arthritis (RA), and systemic lupus erythematosus (SLE). Similar FDA guidelines were subsequently adopted for LASIK. In 2002, the American Academy of Ophthalmology (AAO) issued guidelines stating that antecedent and stable systemic disease is a relative contraindication to LRS, and uncontrolled systemic disease is an absolute contraindication. Notably, the recommendations of the FDA and the AAO were not based on clinical studies and outcomes, but rather on the known ocular complications of these disorders as well as the documented outcomes of nonlaser ocular surgery in such patients—surgery may worsen ocular disease and result in suboptimal outcomes or significant corneal complications including perforations or corneal melt. Further, there is a paucity of literature addressing such questions, and opinions vary considerably among our colleagues.

A small, retrospective case series hinted that outcomes among diabetic patients may be worse than in the overall population.[1] However, larger series have shown that outcomes of LRS in patients with stable CVD or DM without ocular involvement are comparable to the average population.[2-4] At the Wilmer Institute, we approach these patients with extreme care and caution.

Henderson BA, Yoo SH. *Curbside Consultation in Refractive and Lens-Based Surgery: 49 Clinical Questions* (pp 3-5)
© 2015 SLACK Incorporated

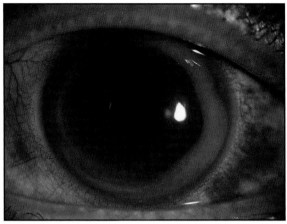

Figure 1-1. Peripheral keratitis after LASIK in a patient with ANA positive and suspicious systemic lupus erythematosus. (Reprinted with permission from Kraig S. Bower, MD.)

We pay careful attention during the preoperative evaluation of each patient to avoid preventable complications and optimize patient outcomes. The potential for a lawsuit is real when there is an unsatisfactory or negative outcome because LRS is off-label, or contraindicated, in these patients. Within the last year, two young patients with underlying CVD underwent LASIK at an outside facility. One presented to our institution with hypopyon-associated uveitis, whereas the other presented with peripheral corneal infiltrates (Figure 1-1).

Diabetes Mellitus

We do not perform LRS on any patient with uncontrolled DM or with diabetic ocular involvement. We require that DM patients be under the care of an internal medicine doctor or an endocrinologist. The DM must be tightly controlled with hemoglobin A1c < 6.5% for at least 6 months. Further, there should not be any evidence of systemic or ocular complications. We perform a thorough slit-lamp exam to exclude any tear film abnormality or insufficiency, subtle corneal epithelial defects, or basement membrane irregularity, and corneal esthesiometry to rule out neuropathy. Finally, we do a careful dilated fundus examination to look for any evidence of diabetic retinopathy or papillopathy.

Collagen Vascular Diseases

We exclude any patient with moderate or severe disease, as well as patients who need a multi-drug regimen to control disease. We demand that an immunologist or a rheumatologist actively care for CVD patients and perform the entire workup. There should be no evidence of systemic activity or flare-up for a minimum of 6 months. There should be no history of ocular involvement. The patient must be cleared for surgery by a rheumatologist, a uveitis specialist, or both. At minimum, the patient should have a documented negative workup for Sjögren's syndrome. We then perform a thorough ocular history and physical exam, including a careful slit-lamp exam to exclude tear film abnormality or insufficiency. We normally perform a Schirmer's test as well as tear break-up time tests. We evaluate for decreased tear film, superficial punctate keratopathy, punctate epithelial erosions, or corneal filaments. We look for signs of uveitis, episcleritis, or scleritis. Finally, we do a careful dilated fundus examination to look for any evidence of retinopathy or vascular abnormality.

Once a patient meets our stringent criteria, we have a detailed and documented discussion of the benefits, risks, and alternatives of LRS. Further, we extensively discuss the patient's underlying disease, potential ocular involvement of the disease, and potential perioperative complications secondary to the disease that are not present in an otherwise healthy patient. Furthermore, we disclose that the long-term outcome of LRS is unknown and that such a procedure is off-label in this patient population according to FDA guidelines.

If a patient still wants LRS, we favor LASIK over PRK. LASIK has a faster healing time in patients with potentially compromised corneal epithelial cells and carries lower risk of stromal haze and scarring in patients with an underlying inflammatory disorder. Further, we favor femtosecond laser-assisted flap creation over the manual keratome to lessen the risk of epithelial shearing.

During the postoperative period, we follow these patients according to our regular schedule with special attention to dry eye disease, corneal haze, epithelial disease, and uveitis.

Conclusion

A patient with an underlying systemic disorder is never ideal for LRS. However, with well-controlled and mild disease and no ocular involvement, patients who are not on a multidrug regimen may be suitable candidates if they meet our stringent criteria. A detailed and documented discussion, including FDA and AAO guidelines, should take place and informed consent obtained. Each patient should be addressed on a case-by-case basis.

References

1. Fraunfelder FW, Rich LF. Laser-assisted in situ keratomileusis complications in diabetes mellitus. *Cornea.* 2002;21(3):246-248.
2. Cobo-Soriano R, Beltrán J, Baviera J. LASIK outcomes in patients with underlying systemic contraindications: A preliminary study. *Ophthalmology.* 2006;113(7):1118.e1-8.
3. Alió JL, Artola A, Belda JI, et al. LASIK in patients with rheumatic diseases: A pilot study. *Ophthalmology.* 2005;112(11):1948-1954.
4. Halkiadakis I, Belfair N, Gimbel HV. Laser in situ keratomileusis in patients with diabetes. *J Cataract Refract Surg.* 2005;31(10):1895-1898.

QUESTION

Should I Perform Refractive Surgery in Patients With a History of Strabismus?

Gabriela L. Pagano, MD and Ofelia Brugnoli de Pagano, MD

The answer is yes, if you know what may happen. The problem we most frequently encounter is that of the myopic patient who undergoes refractive surgery and later complains, "I see perfectly at distance, but up close, it becomes more difficult and I get tired!" This is due to accommodative and convergence insufficiency and happens mostly in myopes who were undercorrected before surgery or who previously removed their spectacles to read. They did not need to accommodate to see near objects before, and now that they are emmetropic, they do. In this group of patients, if the problem persists after 1 month, orthoptic exercises are indicated. This therapy usually works well and quickly.

The most feared problem is diplopia. First, we need to rule out monocular diplopia due to intraoperative complications or technical problems, such as decentered ablation, incomplete flaps, buttonholes, and reduced optical zone, among others.[1]

Binocular diplopia is due to a loss of binocular vision, and this usually results from a decompensation of preexisting strabismus after the refractive procedure.

It would be ideal to perform a sensorimotor exam with and without optical correction on every patient to look for undiagnosed deviations prior to a refractive procedure. We recommend at least alternate cover/uncover testing, a stereopsis exam, and looking for asymmetry in red reflex to avoid surprises in the postoperative period. A cycloplegic refraction is always suggested.

In myopic patients with esodeviation, the deviation may worsen after a refractive procedure, depending on the accommodative component of the strabismus. If the patient is older than 35 to 40 years, the influence is less because of the loss of accommodation with aging. We therefore recommend correcting the least myopic refraction possible (the least negative refraction that does not reduce corrected distance visual acuity [CDVA]) and checking the influence of the intended correction on the deviation. Diplopia may develop after surgery in these patients and strabismus surgery may be necessary afterwards (Figure 2-1).

Henderson BA, Yoo SH. *Curbside Consultation in Refractive and Lens-Based Surgery: 49 Clinical Questions* (pp 7-10)
© 2015 SLACK Incorporated

Figure 2-1. Esotropia of 25 Δ (A) that worsens to 35 Δ with myopic spectacles (B). Orthophoria after myopic refractive surgery followed by strabismus surgery (C).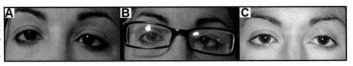

Figure 2-2. Intermittent exotropia of 25 Δ without optical correction (A) in patient with myopic anisometropy (OD –0.50 –1.75 × 175 degrees D and OS –5.00 –1.00 × 0 degrees D) improves to 12 Δ exophoria with spectacles (B). Good ocular alignment after refractive surgery (C).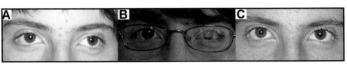

On the other hand, myopes with exotropia may improve their angle of deviation with the refractive procedure[2] as they would with spectacles or contact lenses. In this case, we recommend fully correcting the cycloplegic myopic refraction, or even slightly overcorrecting myopic patients with intermittent exotropia, targeting for the most negative refraction that does not reduce CDVA. This negative correction stimulates accommodation and convergence, which is why intermittent exotropia improves (Figure 2-2). If an angle of deviation remains, it may require treatment with strabismus surgery.

Hyperopic patients with esodeviation may improve their strabismus after a refractive surgery, as they might with the use of spectacles or contact lenses, because fully correcting hyperopia eliminates the patient's need to accommodate and therefore converge. Patients with fully or partially refractive accommodative esotropia are the best candidates for a refractive procedure[3] (Figure 2-3). Again, the improvement in the angle of deviation will depend on the accommodative component of the strabismus. In this group of patients, attempt to correct the more positive refraction (maximum tolerated cycloplegic refraction) that does not reduce CDVA. We have performed hyperopic LASIK in accommodative esotropia patients with refraction of more than +6 diopters (D) with good results and patient satisfaction, but if it helps you sleep better, you can set your cut-off point at +6 D because most refractive accommodative esotropia patients will fall in the +2 to +5 D range.

Patients with hyperopia and exodeviation may worsen with a refractive procedure (Figure 2-4). This is the group of strabismic patients for whom refractive surgery would be least recommended. It can be performed, but the patient should be informed of the possibility of needing strabismus surgery afterwards.

How much can patients improve their angle of deviation? A lot, a little, or nothing, depending on the accommodative component of the strabismus, which is more significant in younger patients. This can be measured with alternate cover/uncover testing and prisms while the patient is wearing the intended optical correction.

If the refractive correction does not change the angle, improves it a little, or worsens it, it is very important to know and to explain to the patient that he or she will need to undergo refractive surgery, and later strabismus surgery. You should perform the refractive procedure first in order to have healthy conjunctiva for the suction ring and because we obtain better results in correcting the angle of deviation when basing the strabismus surgery on the post-LASIK alignment. Furthermore, the better visual acuity improves binocular vision, which results in a more stable orthotropia.

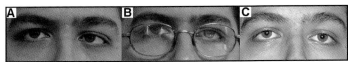

Figure 2-3. Refractive accommodative esotropia of 25 Δ without optical correction (A) and 6 Δ with spectacles (OD +3.00 D and OS +3.50 D) (B). Successful ocular alignment after hyperopic refractive surgery (C).

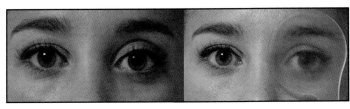

Figure 2-4. Hyperope with intermittent exotropia. If we perform refractive surgery, the deviation may become permanent.

Permanent or manifest strabismus is not a contraindication for a refractive procedure, but a preoperative sensorimotor exam with and without optical correction is mandatory. The target is most frequently emmetropia in both eyes, taking into account the rules previously described.

In most cases, we discourage performing monovision in patients with strabismus. Patients with intermittent strabismus are particularly at risk of losing the ability to fuse images, resulting in diplopia.[1]

Patients with previous strabismus surgery can also be candidates for a refractive procedure. In most cases, you should strive for emmetropia and verify the effect of the intended correction in the angle of deviation. You can also play with slight over- or undercorrections according to the previous guidelines.

Patients with strabismus and anisometropia may benefit from refractive surgery, as these patients can be managed only with contact lenses or a refractive procedure. When performing refractive surgery in amblyopic eyes, if both eyes have a refractive defect, it is important to treat both eyes and aim for emmetropia. Improvement in amblyopia will depend on the patient's age and the type and magnitude of the refractive error—younger patients and myopes achieve better results. It is important to know that only the refractive amblyopia can improve, not the strabic amblyopia. If the patient does not have central fixation, do not do refractive surgery.

Regarding nystagmus, contact lenses and refractive surgery are helpful because they improve foveation of images. Improvement in lines of visual acuity has been observed after refractive surgery. It is helpful to use the eye tracker or, if the laser does not have a tracking system, to keep the eye fixed with the microkeratome suction ring at low or no pressure.

Tips to keep in mind:

- Always ask patients for a history of strabismus or occasional eye deviations because they may not disclose it spontaneously.

- Screen the patient for a possible undiagnosed strabismus: cover/uncover testing (especially with the intended optical correction) for far and near distances, stereopsis exam to assess binocularity, and asymmetry in the red reflex.

- If you have doubts, try first with contact lenses (with the refraction you intend to correct) for at least 1 week and see what happens.

- Esotropia with myopia can get worse.

- Exotropia with hyperopia can get worse.

- Esotropia with hyperopia can get better.

- Exotropia with myopia can get better.
- These rules also apply to patients with previous strabismus surgery.
- If a combined procedure is planned, it is better to perform the refractive surgery first, and the strabismus surgery later.

If your patient develops diplopia after surgery, it is not the end of the world. There is always a strabismus surgeon to fix it. In these cases, we prefer adjustable sutures for more accurate results.

Acknowledgments

The authors wish to acknowledge Alejandro Navas, MD, MSc for his helpful insights and critical review of the chapter.

References

1. Kushner BJ, Kowal L. Diplopia after refractive surgery: Occurrence and prevention. *Arch Ophthalmol.* 2003;121:315-321.
2. Minnal VR, Rosenberg JB. Refractive surgery: A treatment and a cause of strabismus. *Curr Opin Ophthalmol.* 2011;22:222-225.
3. Brugnoli de Pagano OM, Pagano GL. Laser in situ keratomileusis for the treatment of refractive accommodative esotropia. *Ophthalmology.* 2012;119:159-163.

MY PATIENT IS A 25-YEAR-OLD LATENT HYPEROPE. HIS MANIFEST REFRACTION IS +2.0 D, BUT AFTER CYCLOPLEGIA IT IS +4.0 D. WHICH REFRACTION SHOULD I TREAT?

Alain Saad, MD and Damien Gatinel, MD

Understanding hyperopia, performing a good cycloplegic and noncycloplegic refraction, and considering patients' visual needs are essential to obtain satisfying results in hyperopia laser correction. Hyperopia is a common condition, affecting approximately 10% of adults in the United States, and refers to light striking the retina before converging at its focal point (Figure 3-1). It creates difficulty when focusing on close objects, but depending on severity, can also affect distance vision.

Hyperopia can be divided into three parts based on refraction: manifest, latent, and total. *Manifest hyperopia* is that which cannot be overcome by the accommodative muscles; it is measured by the amount of plus sphere that produces best vision and corresponds to the minimal power of spectacle correction required to see clearly. *Latent hyperopia* is the amount of plus sphere measured above the manifest hyperopia after paralysis of the muscles that control accommodation with cycloplegic eye drops; in other words, it is the amount of hyperopia corrected by the physiologic tone of the ciliary muscle. *Total hyperopia* is the sum of latent and manifest hyperopia. For example, a hyperope who sees 20/40 uncorrected may require +2.00 sphere to see 20/20 (this means the patient has 2.00 diopters [D] of manifest hyperopia). After cycloplegic drops are used, the patient requires an additional +2.00 sphere to see 20/20, for a total of +4.00 (this represents +2.00 D of latent hyperopia and +4.00 D of total hyperopia).

Treatment

There is no universal approach to the surgical treatment of hyperopia. Each situation is unique, and patient characteristics such as age, presence of symptoms, amount of hyperopia, and difference

Henderson BA, Yoo SH. *Curbside Consultation in Refractive and Lens-Based Surgery: 49 Clinical Questions* (pp 11-13)
© 2015 SLACK Incorporated

Figure 3-1. Light striking the retina before converging at its focal point in a hyperopic eye.

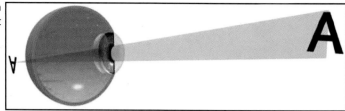

Figure 3-2. Optical zone (ZO) and transitional zone (ZT) in a hyperopic ablation. The photoablated stromal bed is shown in purple and the transition zone in blue. Ablation thickness is zero in the center and maximal at the periphery of the optical zone.

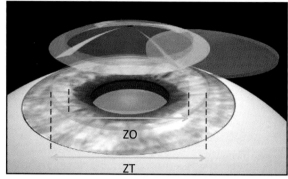

between total and manifest hyperopia should be considered. In addition, the patient's vision needs must be discussed and understood.

In this particular 25-year-old patient with +2.00 D of manifest refraction, the goals of our treatment are to reduce the accommodative demand and to provide clear and comfortable vision. We first search for symptoms such as blur at near, visual discomfort under strenuous visual demand, eye strain headaches, or fatigue after performing work at close range. In the absence of these signs, and if the patient's own correction is +2.00 D, we would plan the laser correction according to this manifest correction (+2 D). The goal of the surgery is to provide the patient with the best uncorrected distance and near visual acuity, while maintaining visual comfort.

It is well known that many patients with latent hyperopia do not tolerate the full correction indicated under cycloplegia. These patients usually have an excellent distance visual acuity and prefer not to lose it. Correcting the total hyperopia (+4 D in this example) will lead to a transient, suboptimal result, especially for distance visual acuity. This may persist for the first postoperative months (period of adaptation/relaxation of the accommodation). The "wow" effect of the LASIK procedure disappears, and even if a thorough explanation of this transient adaptation period is discussed with the patient preoperatively, few patients really understand or accept it.

Most of today's scanning laser systems used in the LASIK procedures can safely and effectively perform low, moderate, and high hyperopic corrections. The "spot scanning" or "flying spot" laser platforms allow correction of hyperopia over a larger optical zone and transition zone up to 9 mm (Figure 3-2). The larger stromal bed exposures obtained with the femtosecond laser flap cuts have significantly improved the long-term refractive stability of hyperopic treatments. Depending on the laser platform used and the individual results of the surgeon, the appropriate nomogram should be applied to achieve a +2.00 D correction, while allowing for the regression that may occur postoperatively.

In 5 to 10 years, the patient's latent hyperopia may decrease and his or her manifest hyperopia may increase due to decreasing accommodative amplitudes. Thus, the patient should be made aware of the possibility of needing an enhancement in about 10 years.

An alternative approach is to prescribe glasses preoperatively with 1 additional diopter above the manifest refraction (3 D in this case) in order to reduce the latent hyperopia. This approach is justified if the patient complains of headache or fatigue while working at near, or if his or her vision needs at near are much greater than at distance. In such cases, the patient should understand the role of the "overcorrected" glasses and the need for some time to tolerate it. Follow-up at 1 or 2 months is needed to ensure the patient's tolerance, evaluate visual symptoms, and remeasure latent and manifest refraction. If well tolerated, the latent hyperopia will likely decrease by about 1 D. Thus, a hyperopic ablation of 3 D may be performed.

Bibliography

Benjamin WJ, Borish IM. *Borish's Clinical Refraction*. 2nd ed. St. Louis: Butterworth Heinemann; 2006:9-11.

Lukenda A, Martinović ZK, Kalauz M. Excimer laser correction of hyperopia, hyperopic and mixed astigmatism: Past, present, and future. *Acta Clin Croat*. 2012;51(2):299-304.

Sher NA. Hyperopic refractive surgery. *Curr Opin Ophthalmol*. 2001;12(4):304-308.

Sorsby A. The functional anomalies. *Modern Ophthalmology*. Philadelphia: JB Lippincott; 1972:9-29.

4

WHAT ARE THE CORNEAL PACHYMETRY THRESHOLDS FOR PERFORMING LASIK, PRK, OR NO LASER VISION CORRECTION AT ALL?

J. Bradley Randleman, MD

Patients with low preoperative corneal thickness are at increased risk of developing ectasia after photorefractive keratectomy (PRK) or LASIK.[1] While a variety of different cut-off values have been presented over the years (with 500 microns frequently considered the lower limit for LASIK), there is no established pachymetry minimum to prevent postoperative ectasia. Fueling the debate, there are reports of patients with good postoperative outcomes with preoperative pachymetry less than 500 microns,[2] despite population analyses reporting that thin corneas are at increased risk.[1] Even so, we have sufficient data to determine useful guidelines for minimum pachymetry, especially when considered within the context of corneal topographic patterns, patient age, and regional pachymetry measurements.

Corneal thinning is a hallmark feature of corneal ectatic disorders, including keratoconus. Population-based analyses show significant differences in corneal thickness between ectatic and normal corneas. Various studies have found that average central corneal thickness in the normal population is approximately 540 to 560 microns with a standard deviation of 30 to 50 microns; thus, 99% of normal corneas are between 450 and 650 microns thick. Using these values, 450 microns seems reasonable as a lower threshold for any laser vision correction, regardless of other patient variables.[1] For measurements between 450 and 500, the picture is less clear.

There is significant overlap in central pachymetry of normal and ectatic populations, and considered alone, it is a limited predictor of disease within the normal range (±1 standard deviation). Using available data, a patient with central pachymetry under 480 microns has less than a 3% chance of being a normal candidate. Most clinicians, therefore, do not routinely offer LASIK to these individuals; however, surface ablation may be a reasonable alternative for patients with no other suspicious findings.

Henderson BA, Yoo SH. *Curbside Consultation in Refractive and Lens-Based Surgery: 49 Clinical Questions* (pp 15-17) © 2015 SLACK Incorporated

Figure 4-1. Scanning-slit beam composite image of the keratometry and corneal thickness maps for the right (top) and left (bottom) eye of the same patient. Note the topographic pattern asymmetry between eyes and abnormal relational thickness profiles, with abnormally low thickness progression in the temporal direction for both eyes.

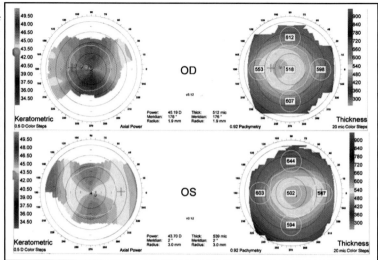

Figure 4-2. Corneal thickness spatial profile generated by the Pentacam Scheimpflug imaging system (Oculus, Inc). As viewed from left to right, the red line follows thickness progression for this eye. Note that the red line deviates significantly below the appropriate line, indicating an abnormal ratio between central and peripheral thickness.

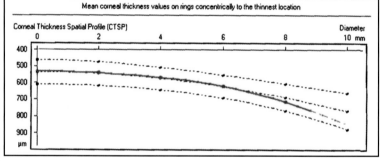

Evaluating corneal thickness independently has some value, but much more can be gained when pachymetry is considered within the context of other preoperative testing, especially corneal topography. Ectatic corneas display focal areas of both steepening and thinning. The order in which these findings become manifest is a matter of great debate; nevertheless, if subtle topographic abnormalities exist, including asymmetric patterns within and between eyes combined with subtle thinning, this is concerning for increased ectasia risk.

Topographic pattern evaluation and corneal thickness should be considered in the context of patient age. Because corneal thinning and warpage are progressive by nature in ectatic disease, findings in younger patients may be less dramatic. Young patient age is an established risk factor for ectasia, likely for this reason.[1] Young patients with slightly thinner corneas and subtle topographic asymmetries should be considered higher risk for laser vision correction unless more advanced testing metrics can determine them to be normal.

A variety of technologies have been developed to supplement current screening strategies but they will require validation of their efficacy. Scanning slit beam and Scheimpflug imaging devices can provide anterior and posterior corneal elevation data. Perhaps more important, regional corneal thickness values are now available using scanning slit (Figure 4-1), Scheimpflug (Figure 4-2),[3] and high-resolution anterior segment ocular coherence tomography (OCT) (Figure 4-3).[4] All of these technologies display relational corneal thickness (ie, relative progression from central to peripheral

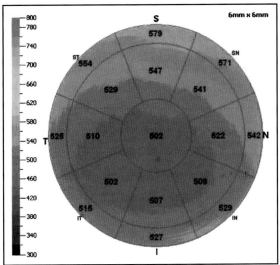

Figure 4-3. OCT image demonstrating a suspicious relational thickness profile. Central thickness is 502 microns and there is minimal increase inferiorly, with peripheral values significantly lower than the corresponding areas superiorly.

corneal thickness measurements). Normal corneas are thinnest centrally and thicken predictably and robustly to the periphery, while eyes with ectatic disease do not thicken as greatly or as uniformly. Specific regional relationships have yet to be determined, especially in ectasia-suspect eyes, but this metric has shown promise in patient evaluation and should be considered, especially in borderline individuals. The Ocular Response Analyzer (Reichert) has also been touted for its ability to directly measure corneal biomechanics and theoretically lessen the importance of indirect measures such as thickness or curvature. To date, however, reported efficacy of this technology is limited because normal and ectatic populations overlap significantly. It may play a role in adjunctive testing for borderline individuals.

Conclusion

While definitive pachymetry values that apply to all individuals remain elusive, it seems prudent to use 450 microns as a relative cut-off for any laser vision correction and 480 microns or thereabouts as a cut-off for most LASIK cases. All patients require extensive evaluation beyond central corneal pachymetry, including advanced topographic analysis with results interpreted in the context of patient age, and regional and relational corneal thickness considered, at least for borderline cases.

References

1. Randleman JB, Woodward M, Lynn MJ, Stulting RD. Risk assessment for ectasia after corneal refractive surgery. *Ophthalmology.* 2008;115:37-50.
2. Kymionis GD, Bouzoukis D, Diakonis V, et al. Long-term results of thin corneas after refractive laser surgery. *Am J Ophthalmol.* 2007;144:181-185.
3. Ambrosio R Jr, Caiado AL, Guerra FP, et al. Novel pachymetric parameters based on corneal tomography for diagnosing keratoconus. *J Refract Surg.* 2011;27:753-758.
4. Li Y, Meisler DM, Tang M, et al. Keratoconus diagnosis with optical coherence tomography pachymetry mapping. *Ophthalmology.* 2008;115:2159-2166.

QUESTION

5

AFTER RADIAL KERATOTOMY, SHOULD I PERFORM PRK OR LASIK SURGERY?

Ramon Coral Ghanem, MD, PhD and Vinícius Coral Ghanem, MD, PhD

Radial keratotomy (RK), a procedure in which 90%- to 95%-thickness radial incisions are made in the paracentral and peripheral cornea using a diamond-bladed micrometer knife, was the most widely used refractive surgical procedure to correct myopia during the 1980s and early 1990s. With this technique, the radial incisions cause biomechanical weakening of the peripheral cornea, resulting in peripheral steepening and compensatory central flattening. In most cases, over decades, progressive weakening causes hyperopic shift, the main complication of this surgery. Excessive central flattening reduces optical quality of the cornea, creates positive spherical aberration, and decreases contrast sensitivity.

The management of refractive errors after RK is unique and challenging. These corneas are usually very flat and irregular with different biomechanical and healing responses than virgin corneas, producing worse visual and refractive outcomes. LASIK has been widely used and, despite its good short-term efficacy, many flap-related complications have been described, including opening of the RK incisions during flap lift, diffuse lamellar keratitis, and epithelial ingrowth.[1] Another important concern when performing LASIK after RK is possible augmentation of the inherent corneal structural instability, potentially leading to iatrogenic corneal ectasia. In our experience, photorefractive keratectomy (PRK) is the best option to treat both residual myopia and hyperopia after RK, which is much more common and will be described later in this chapter.[2,3] Clinically significant corneal haze, the main concern in these patients, is uncommon when mitomycin C (MMC) is used.[3] An alternative to PRK is purse-string suturing, a continuous intrastromal suture of the spaces between the radial incisions. This technique is usually restricted to higher hyperopic corrections because of its low predictability, poor long-term stability, and technical complexity. Hyperopic phakic intraocular lenses may be implanted when the cornea is regular but too thin for

Henderson BA, Yoo SH. *Curbside Consultation in Refractive and Lens-Based Surgery: 49 Clinical Questions* (pp 19-21)
© 2015 SLACK Incorporated

Figure 5-1. Consecutive hyperopia and irregular astigmatism after RK treated with corneal wavefront-guided PRK with adjunctive MMC 0.02%. A 46-year-old female underwent an uncomplicated 8-incision RK with 4 arcuate incisions in 1988 for myopic astigmatism. In November 2007, she was evaluated for complaints of decreased near and distance vision. At that time, uncorrected visual acuity was 20/200 and her cycloplegic refraction was +5.00 – 1.00 x 120 degrees (20/25–). (A) Pre- and (B) postoperative tangential topography and (C) pre- and (D) postoperative (at 2 years) corneal wave front analysis. Two years after PRK, her uncorrected visual acuity was 20/30 and her refraction was –0.25 – 0.50 x 140 degrees (20/25+). Note the improved corneal shape and decreased corneal aberrations.

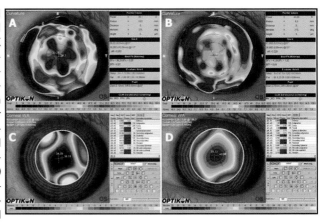

Figure 5-2. Ectatic radial incision seen on (A) direct illumination and (B) retroillumination (arrows). (C) Corneal OCT reveals widened radial incision with downward proliferation of corneal epithelium (arrowhead).

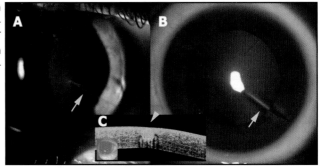

PRK, the refractive error is significant, and the corrected visual acuity is satisfactory. Note that the anterior chamber is usually deep in these previously myopic patients.

Photorefractive Keratectomy Pearls

Patient Selection

PRK can be indicated for patients with hyperopia or hyperopic astigmatism with spherical equivalent of up to +8.00 D and astigmatism of up to –6.0 D. In our recently published series of 61 eyes followed for 2 years, the patients that had worse preoperative corrected distance visual acuity were the ones with higher ametropia and corneal flattening; these patients experienced a greater gain of lines after corneal wavefront-guided PRK, mainly due to corneal steepening and decrease of corneal aberrations (Figure 5-1).[3] Patients with thin corneas (usually central pachymetry < 490 µm) and suspected keratoconus should not be operated on. Ectatic or fairly widened radial incisions should be sutured before PRK (Figure 5-2). We usually wait 6 months after suturing to perform the laser.

Surgical Technique

Because most corneas after RK suffer from significant high-order aberrations and some degree of irregular astigmatism, customized photoablations are usually appropriate. Total wavefront analysis, however, has limited value in very irregular corneas. Most wavefront devices are unable to acquire reproducible measurements of ocular aberrations in these cases; furthermore, the exam is limited to the pupil size and can be influenced by accommodation. Topography, in contrast, has high precision and reproducibility in the central 8 to 9 mm of the cornea, allowing evaluation of the curvature, irregularities, and anterior surface wavefront errors. Therefore, we consider topography-guided or corneal wavefront-guided ablations more suitable for treating post-RK refractive errors.

Important surgical steps include the following:

- Cyclotorsion control, either manually using limbal marks or automated by the eye tracker.

- Mechanical centripetal epithelial removal in the photoablation area, in order to avoid opening RK incisions. We do not recommend transepithelial treatment because the epithelium is much thicker centrally and thinner paracentrally than in the normal population (for whom the transepithelial approach was designed).

- Photoablation aiming at correction of the cycloplegic refraction with a myopic target (usually –1.00) to avoid undercorrection. Nomogram adjustments are recommended. We usually limit ablation to approximately 150 µm.

- MMC 0.2 mg/mL (0.02%) application for 20 or 60 seconds throughout the ablation zone, with longer exposures (40 to 60 seconds) reserved for deeper ablations (> 100 µm), greater number of RK incisions, retreatments, and previously sutured corneas.[3]

Postoperative Care

Therapeutic contact lenses are usually removed after 1 week and loteprednol 0.5% maintained 4 times a day for 1 month. Central haze is rare and peripheral haze up to grade 2+ is common. It usually peaks around 12 months and decreases thereafter. Refraction stability is commonly achieved after 6 months. In our study, a mean hyperopic shift of +0.39 D was observed between 6 and 24 months postoperatively.[3]

References

1. Francesconi CM, Nosé RA, Nosé W. Hyperopic laser-assisted in situ keratomileusis for radial keratotomy induced hyperopia. *Ophthalmology*. 2002;109(3):602-605.
2. Ghanem RC, Ghanem VC, de Souza DC, Kara-José N, Ghanem EA. Customized topography-guided photorefractive keratectomy with the MEL-70 platform and mitomycin C to correct hyperopia after radial keratotomy. *J Refract Surg*. 2008;24(9):911-922.
3. Ghanem RC, Ghanem VC, Ghanem EA, Kara-José N. Corneal wavefront-guided photorefractive keratectomy with mitomycin-C for hyperopia after radial keratotomy: Two-year follow-up. *J Cataract Refract Surg*. 2012;38(4):595-606.

QUESTION

6

ARE THERE SPECIAL CONSIDERATIONS IN THE EVALUATION AND TREATMENT OF PATIENTS WITH HIGH ASTIGMATISM SEEKING LASER VISION CORRECTION?

Afshan Nanji, MD, MPH and Sonia H. Yoo, MD

When evaluating a patient for refractive surgery, the refraction and corneal topography are clearly important parts of the work-up. One factor that may be identified during this evaluation is high astigmatism (more than 2.0 diopters [D]). In the assessment of high astigmatism, one must take into account the degree, symmetry, and regularity of the astigmatism. High astigmatism, when asymmetric, irregular, or associated with decreased pachymetry, suggests an ectatic process that may worsen with refractive surgery. When high astigmatism is detected, closer evaluation of symmetry indices, pachymetry, pachymetric progression, and even corneal biomechanics, if available, is highly recommended to prevent postoperative ectasia.

If, however, the patient is deemed to have high but regular astigmatism, refractive surgery can be performed. Depending on the laser, correction of up to 6.0 D of astigmatism can be corrected. Both photorefractive keratectomy (PRK) and LASIK can have good outcomes in these patients.

In performing any refractive procedure in patients with high astigmatism, a few points must be kept in mind. First, patients should understand that those with more than 1 D of astigmatism are more likely to require retreatment in order to achieve their best-corrected visual acuity.[1] They are more likely to be left with undercorrection of their astigmatism, particularly those with hyperopic astigmatism. Residual astigmatism may decrease uncorrected visual acuity and cause monocular diplopia, particularly at night, and the possibility of retreatment must therefore be discussed. Second, unlike for spherical ablations, cyclotorsional movements induced by monocular fixation and by the change in position that the laser requires can result in decreased correction. Iris registration software, when available, avoids this problem; otherwise, the eye should be marked preoperatively at 3 and 9 o'clock to allow alignment with the reticle and to avoid treating in the incorrect axis.

Henderson BA, Yoo SH. *Curbside Consultation in Refractive and Lens-Based Surgery: 49 Clinical Questions* (pp 23-24)
© 2015 SLACK Incorporated

Traditional treatment of myopic and hyperopic astigmatism uses an elliptical ablation pattern to flatten the steeper meridian of the cornea. This causes the effective optical zone of the ablation to be smaller than the treated area. To avoid an edge effect, a cross cylinder technique can be used in either PRK or LASIK, flattening the steeper meridian and steepening the flatter meridian. By treating both meridians, the ablation profile is smoother. A second strategy for improved outcomes is wavefront-guided treatment, which allows correction of both low- and high-order aberrations. This latter approach has been shown to have better outcomes in PRK in terms of best-corrected and uncorrected postoperative visual acuity for high astigmatism.[2] Also, with PRK, the use of mitomycin C should be considered because treatment of high astigmatism is associated with greater chance of haze.[3]

When high astigmatism results from previous penetrating keratoplasty (PKP), LASIK or PRK may be used. PRK has been found to be safe and effective but, again, the use of mitomycin C is encouraged to prevent haze after treatment of high astigmatism. PRK following PKP is also associated with a high risk of regression. If LASIK is chosen, some surgeons favor a two-step approach, as formation of the LASIK flap alone can change the refraction in these patients. In the first step, the flap is created and lifted, and, in the second visit, the flap is relifted and the ablation performed. The ability to perform LASIK after PKP depends greatly on the graft size because a small flap and small optical zone may increase night glare and halos. For the ablation portion of LASIK or PRK, a wavefront-guided approach may also be useful, given the increase in corneal irregularities. However, wavefront capture may be difficult in these eyes, and topography-guided LASIK can be used to address corneal irregularities and improve higher-order aberrations.

High astigmatism in refractive surgery poses unique challenges in evaluation and treatment; however, careful assessment, counseling, and treatment can produce excellent outcomes in satisfied patients.

References

1. Randleman JB, White AJ, Lynn MJ, Hu MH, Stulting RD. Incidence, outcomes, and risk factors for retreatment after wavefront-optimized ablations with PRK and LASIK. *J Refract Surg.* 2009;25(3):273-276.
2. Sedghipour MR, Sorkhabi R, Mostafaei A. Wavefront-guided versus cross-cylinder photorefractive keratectomy in moderate-to-high astigmatism: A cohort of two consecutive clinical trials. *Clin Ophthalmol.* 2012;6:199-204.
3. Thomas KE, Brunstetter T, Rogers S, Sheridan MV. Astigmatism: Risk factor for postoperative corneal haze in conventional myopic photorefractive keratectomy. *J Cataract Refract Surg.* 2008;34(12):2068-2072.

QUESTION

SHOULD I PERFORM PRK IN PATIENTS WITH FORME FRUSTE KERATOCONUS?

Damien Gatinel, MD

Corneas with subclinical keratoconus are absolutely contraindicated for LASIK surgery. It is less obvious whether topographic suspicion of keratoconus is a strict contraindication for photorefractive keratectomy (PRK). At first glance, one might hesitate to operate on a cornea with potential biomechanical compromise; however, growing evidence suggests that PRK can be a safe and effective therapy for mild myopia and astigmatism in carefully selected patients with forme fruste keratoconus, yielding improved visual function and extended refractive and corneal stability. Early reports have shown stable visual improvement in primary keratoconus with up to 4 years of follow-up.[1]

We became interested in retrospectively analyzing outcomes of PRK on patients with corneas that were identified as at risk of ectasia because we noticed, in our common practice, that corneas classified as keratoconus suspects (KCS) based on computerized Placido analysis did not develop unusual complications or ectatic evolution after surface ablation techniques.

We retrospectively assessed long-term outcomes of PRK in 62 eyes of 42 patients classified as KCS or keratoconus (KC) by the OPD-Scan II corneal navigator (Nidek).[2] These patients had been treated with myopic PRK between 2004 and 2007 at the Rothschild Foundation in Paris, France using the Nidek EC5000 excimer laser. The percentage of similarity to KCS or KC was positive in all 62 eyes and exceeded a 50% similarity score in 30 eyes (48.4%). The mean age was 34.6 ± 15.1 years and the mean spherical equivalent (SE) was -3.96 ± 3.05 diopters (D) (mean sphere, -3.48 ± 3.14 D; mean cylinder, -0.97 ± 0.92 D). The mean central pachymetry was 529.4 ± 32.8 µm (mean thinnest point, 522.1 ± 33.6 µm) and the mean simulated keratometry was 45.75 ± 1.75 D. Mean follow-up was 4.8 ± 1.4 years. The mean magnitude of the SE was -0.53 ± 1.35 D over the follow-up period, with a mean postoperative keratometry of 42.9 ± 2.4 D. Only two patients experienced significant myopic regression requiring glasses. As in previous

Henderson BA, Yoo SH. *Curbside Consultation in Refractive and Lens-Based Surgery: 49 Clinical Questions* (pp 25-26)
© 2015 SLACK Incorporated

reports, whether a physiological variant or subclinical keratoconus, no case of ectasia was reported, and the PRK did not lead to a progression of the suspected KC or any other complication.

The specificity of subclinical KC detection-based Placido topography is not 100%.[3] For some of our patients, an abnormal inferior keratometry minus superior keratometry value (as defined by Rabinowitz[4]) or a steep keratometry (> 47 D) may merely represent a false positive. Some of the included corneas may therefore be physiological variants of normal corneas. Corneas at risk in refractive surgery may be detected with greater sensitivity and specificity by combining tomographic and pachymetric maps and viscoelasticity measurements with the usual Placido topographic index.

Corneal ectasia after PRK has been described in a few case reports wherein affected corneas presented preoperatively with obvious characteristics of KCS[5] or family history of keratoconus. Since 2006, fewer than 10 such reports of ectasia have been reported in the literature.

This low incidence suggests that PRK may not unfavorably influence the evolution of corneas with subclinical keratoconus. In the late 1990s and early 2000s, when topographic screening for forme fruste keratoconus was not as stringent as today, many myopic and astigmatic PRK procedures were performed. Many eyes with forme fruste and subclinical KC likely underwent PRK during that time. If this technique had triggered significant evolution toward ectasia, we would expect to see many more ectatic corneas with a history of PRK. This paradox could even suggest a protective effect from PRK! Inflammation induced by PRK could theoretically halt the progression of keratectasia and induce localized cross-linking, strengthening corneal collagen fibers by linking one polymer chain to another. This questions the interest of the association of riboflavin/UVA CxL to conventional or topography-guided PRK for the treatment of nonprogressive keratoconus.

PRK in eyes with suspected keratoconus based on Placido neural network may be safe and effective for myopia and astigmatism in carefully selected patients. However, treatment must be discussed on a case-by-case basis because limitations exist for steeper and thinner corneas.

References

1. Bilgihan K, Ozdek SC, Konuk O, Akata F, Hasanreisoglu B. Results of photorefractive keratectomy in keratoconus suspects at 4 years. *J Refract Surg*. 2000;16(4):438-443.
2. Guedj M, Saad A, Audureau E, Gatinel D. Photorefractive keratectomy in patients with suspected keratoconus: Five-year follow-up. *J Cataract Refract Surg*. 2013;39(1):66-73.
3. Saad A, Gatinel D. Topographic and tomographic properties of forme fruste keratoconus corneas. *Invest Ophthalmol Vis Sci*. 2010;51(11):5546-5555.
4. Rabinowitz YS. Keratoconus. *Surv Ophthalmol*. 1998;42(4):297-319.
5. Randelman JB, Caster AI, Banning CS, et al. Corneal ectasia after photorefractive keratectomy. *J Cataract Refract Surg*. 2006;32(8):1395-1398.

WHEN SHOULD I PERFORM TOPOGRAPHY-GUIDED OR ABERRATION-GUIDED REFRACTIVE SURGERY?

A.J. Kanellopoulos, MD

I have learned to respect several parameters that may induce aberrations in refractive surgery:

- The LASIK flap
- Excimer ablation decentration
- Excimer ablation irregularities
- Postoperative dry eye
- Blepharitis and meibomian gland dysfunction and disease

Induced flap aberrations have improved over the years due to better flap making (femtosecond lasers) and handling (surgeon experience). Femtosecond laser flaps are more homogeneous in thickness throughout their surface, with a smaller standard deviation of central effective thickness (Figure 8-1).

Using very high frequency ultrasound, we have recently studied several different types of LASIK flaps, including some made with mechanical microkeratomes and some with femtosecond lasers. We found significant differences in overall flap thickness homogeneity that may affect mesopic and scotopic visual function based on symmetry (Figure 8-2).

As little as 100 microns of laser ablation decentration is enough to cause mesopic and scotopic aberrations in myopic ablations.

We currently work with the Wavelight: FS200 femto and EX500 excimer lasers (Alcon). The EX500 employs an impressive 1028-Hz tracker, with an effective 2-msec response time, and produces a smaller deviation of ablations.

My experience mirrors the improvement in tracker and cyclodeviation ability by most lasers, with fewer decentered ablations in patients with large pupils and mesopic and scotopic problems of visual function.

Henderson BA, Yoo SH. *Curbside Consultation in Refractive and Lens-Based Surgery: 49 Clinical Questions* (pp 27-30)
© 2015 SLACK Incorporated

Figure 8-1. Overall correlation between horizontal intended vs achieved flap size. The linear fit regression line and the coefficient of linearity determination (R^2) are shown. The 95% confidence interval (CI) as well as the 95% prediction interval lines are also plotted.[1]

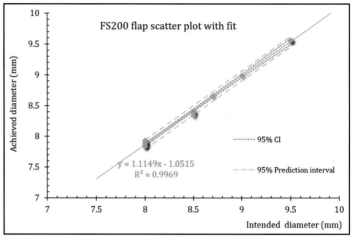

Figure 8-2. Postoperative flap thickness/topographic flap thickness variability for the 3 groups examined.[2]

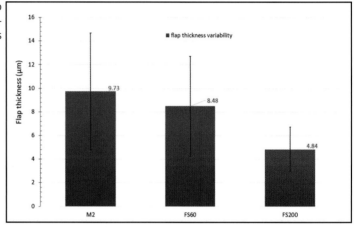

Clinically studying wavefront- and topography-guided ablation over the years has been a fascinating journey, wherein I have had a multitude of experiences from both my European and US practices.

Some of the difficulties in utilizing wavefront analysis of the human eye for treatments are the following:

- Selecting the optimal level of accommodation during the measurement (far vision, intermediate vision, dilated pupil, or cycloplegia)

- Selecting the pupil size where the wavefront will be captured and the treatment delivered

- Selecting the most beneficial among specific Zernike parameters

Applegate has reported that not all Zernike polynomial deviations are "troublesome" for human eyesight; some may enhance contrast ability in some people.

It has been my experience that wavefront-guided treatments, as an enhancement, have benefited many patients by improving mainly spherical aberration—basically, the C12 Zernike polynomial.

One of the arguments for wavefront-optimized treatments (ie, preemptively overtreating the ablation periphery to reduce spherical aberration) vs wavefront-guided treatments is that normal eyes usually do not have high-order aberrations and it wouldn't make sense to employ

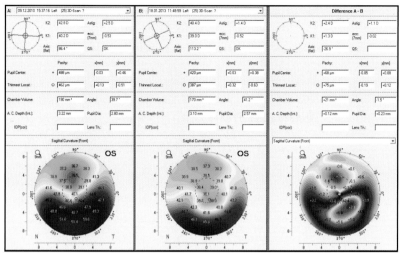

Figure 8-3. This is an example of a post-LASIK ectasia I treated with the Athens Protocol (topography-guided partial PRK and CXL): The left is the ectasia stage, the middle is current (2 years post-AP), and the right image shows pre- minus post-LASIK, showing the dramatic and specific normalization of the corneal irregularity.

wavefront-guided treatment because this could possibly decrease some and increase other higher aberrations due to capture and/or delivery error.

The advantage of topography-guided treatments, in my opinion, is that the corneal surface is affected minimally by pupil size or different levels of accommodation and therefore may offer a more stable medium to be imaged and treated. I have used the Wavelight topography-guided platform with very reproducible results, even in treating significant irregularities. Topography data can be introduced by 2 diagnostic devices:

1. A Placido disc device (the Topolyzer or currently the Vario [Alcon]) offering data even in "cloudy" corneas.
2. Pentacam (OCULUS Optikgeräte GmbH) (tomography/Scheimflug)-based platform (the Oculyzer and currently the Oculyzer II [WaveLight]) offers better imaging of the center of the cornea but is potentially affected by opacities in the cornea.

Topography-guided treatments of irregular corneas (eg, with scars, previously decentered ablations, or ectasia) are not yet perfected for calculating the spherical equivalent change that the treatment will induce because they are based on corneal curvature and do not "see" the axial length of the eye. In my experience, topography-guided treatments appear far more useful clinically than wavefront-guided because they can be used in over 95% of cases, even with extremely irregular corneas, keratoconus, and post-LASIK ectasia (Figure 8-3).

What Do I Do in My Practice?

I employ wavefront, topography, cornea tomography (Pentacam) and axial length measurements in standard preoperative evaluation data for LASIK candidates.

- For myopes, I employ wavefront-optimized treatment.
- For myopic eyes with aberrations measured over 0.4, I consider a wavefront-guided primary treatment.
- For hyperopia, I use a primary, topography-guided treatment, using the same platform, with a 9.5-mm flap at 130-micron depth. The topography-guided treatment aims to center the hyperopic ablation at the visual axis, which is typically nasal to the pupil center (angle kappa).

- For keratoconus and ectasia, I use the Athens Protocol, a combination of a topography-guided excimer surface normalization of the cornea and high fluence CXL (Avedro).

- If a retreatment is necessary, I consider all custom modalities: wavefront-guided, topography-guided, and ray-tracing.

Conclusion

Refractive surgery currently offers very robust choices in technologies and techniques. Many of these have crossover potential as helpful tools for corneal reconstructive work. Nevertheless, I believe that the ultimate treatment tool is the surgeon. To have successful outcomes requires broad knowledge, thorough assessment, and critical judgment, not only of the specific biologic parameters, but also understanding the desires, needs, and expectations of patients.

Acknowledgments

I wish to acknowledge some of the earliest proponents of these modalities: Theo Seiler, Michael Mrochen, Ray Applegate, Steven Schalhorn, and Ron Krueger.

Bibliography

Applegate RA, Sarver EJ, Khemsara V. Are all aberrations equal? *J Refract Surg.* 2002;18(5):S556-S562.

Kanellopoulos AJ. Long-term comparison of sequential vs. same day simultaneous collagen cross-linking (CXL) and topography-guided PRK (TgPRK) for treatment of keratoconus (KCN). *J Refract Surg.* 2009;25(9):S812-S818.

Kanellopoulos AJ, Asimellis G. Flap parameter accuracy, opaque bubble layer and skip-line study in femtosecond laser assisted LASIK. A novel technique of assessment. *Clin Ophthalmol.* 2013;7:343-351.

Kanellopoulos AJ, Asimellis G. High frequency ultrasound comparison of topographic central, paracentral and peripheral LASIK flap thickness variability, in flaps created by a mechanical microkeratome (M2) and two different femtosecond lasers (FS60 and FS200). *Clin Ophthalmol.* 2013;7:675-683.

Kanellopoulos AJ, Binder PS. Collagen cross-linking (CCL) with sequential topography-guided PRK. A temporizing alternative for keratoconus to penetrating keratoplasty. *Cornea.* 2007;26:891-895.

SECTION II

SURGICAL PROCEDURE

HOW SHOULD I CENTER MY ABLATION IN PATIENTS WITH A LARGE ANGLE KAPPA?

Samuel Arba Mosquera, PhD, MSc

The *angle kappa* is the angular distance between the visual and the pupillary axes (Figure 9-1). It is strongly related to (and often mistaken for) the angles alpha (optical to visual axis) and lambda (pupillary axis to line-of-sight).[1]

Because there is significant variability in the values of these angles among different patients, but strong specular symmetry between two eyes of the same patient, it is difficult to conclude which centration technique is superior. Further, some diagnostic systems may report these angles in degrees (as angular distance) but more report them as offset distances (in mm or μm) at the corneal plane (Figure 9-2).

There are several approaches to managing large angle kappa.[2] The most common of these is to determine the coaxial corneal light reflex (first Purkinje image); however, the coaxial light reflex will be seen differently depending on surgeon eye dominance, surgeon eye balance, and the stereopsis angle of the microscope. To account for this, the LadarVision platform (Alcon) uses a coaxial photograph to determine the coaxial light reflex, eliminating the variable of the surgeon's focus, and the MEL80 platform (Zeiss-Meditec) proposes using the surgeon's contralateral eye to determine the corneal coaxial light reflex (patient's OD determined through surgeon's OS and vice versa) to reduce parallax. I prefer to take the numeric values of the offset distance at the corneal plane and with them shift the optical axis of the ablation to the coordinates of the corneal vertex. This improves objectivity (the values are measured from an instantaneous snapshot), robustness (several measurements can be taken and averaged), and concordance (the values from the diagnosis are taken directly from the diagnostic device [no conversion whatsoever] to the laser).

Considering this, for sphere, cylinder, and axis values taken from manifest refraction, the most appropriate centering reference is the visual axis (corneal vertex or corneal coaxial light reflex). High-order aberrations (eg, in wavefront-guided treatments) are described for a reference point in

Henderson BA, Yoo SH. *Curbside Consultation in Refractive and Lens-Based Surgery: 49 Clinical Questions* (pp 33-35)
© 2015 SLACK Incorporated

Figure 9-1. Reference axes of the human eye. (Modified from Arbelaez MC, Vidal C, Arba Mosquera S. Clinical outcomes of corneal vertex versus central pupil references with aberration-free ablation strategies and LASIK. *Invest Ophthalmol Vis Sci.* 2008;49:5287-5294. © Association for Research in Vision and Ophthalmology.)

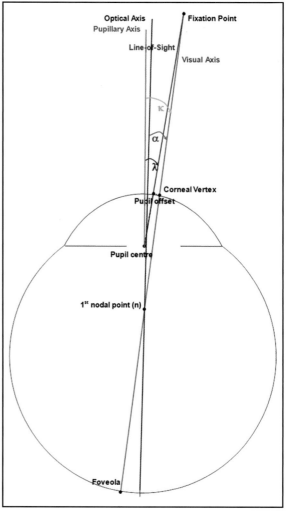

Figure 9-2. Example of a large angle kappa reported as offset distance (in mm) at the corneal plane. In our experience, the pupillary offset averages 0.2 mm, which appears to be large enough to account for differences in ocular aberrations, but not enough to correlate this difference in ocular aberrations with functional vision. We can broadly categorize angle kappa as being small (below 5 degrees or 200 μm) or large (more than 5 degrees or 200 μm).

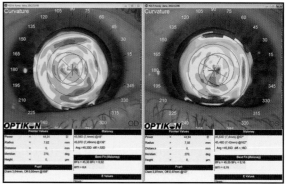

the center of the entrance pupil. For those, the most appropriate centering reference is the entrance pupil as measured in the diagnosis.

As a general principle, be attentive to the magnitude and direction of the angle kappa (small vs large, but also nasal vs temporal, inferior vs superior, and symmetry between eyes). Use offsets or determine the corneal coaxial light reflex for large angle kappa several times to assess consistency. Perform ablations close to the visual axis by using offset values, but use pupil center when in doubt. Moreover, in patients with corneal problems such as keratoconus/keratectasia, post-LASIK (pupil-centered), corneal warping induced by contact lenses, and other diseases causing irregularity of the anterior corneal surface, the corneal vertex and apex may shift. In those cases, the pupil center is probably more stable.

It may also be of interest to refer the corneal and/or ocular wavefront measurements to the visual axis or corneal vertex. This can be done easily for corneal wavefront analysis because pupil boundaries impose no limitation. However, it is not as easy for ocular wavefront analysis because only the portion of the cornea above the entrance pupil is responsible for foveal vision.

Many assume that these two strategies (pupil center and corneal vertex) are opposite concepts, and that surgeons must decide between them. Some opt for an ablation center between pupil center and corneal vertex as a sort of compromise. One system now offers an asymmetric offset approach[2] demonstrating that the strategies are complementary and can be implemented together. This utilizes eye-tracker functionality, with pupil center as the reference for the center of the ablation and corneal vertex as the optical axis of the ablation.

Ablating on the visual axis (corneal vertex) should result in less asymmetric aberration (coma and trefoil), and avoid undercorrections and nomograms by placing the peak of the ablation on or near the visual axis. This is confirmed by studies that also claim superiority of visual axis references over pupil-based ones.[3,4]

References

1. Thibos LN. How to Measure Chromatic Aberration and Locate Useful Reference Axes of the Human Eye - 31 slides presented at OSA '95 meeting in Portland, OR in September 1995. Available at: http://www.opt.indiana.edu/people/faculty/thibos/ABLNTOSA95/slide01.html
2. Arba Mosquera S, Ewering T. New asymmetric centration strategy combining pupil and corneal vertex information for ablation procedures in refractive surgery: Theoretical background. *J Refract Surg.* 2012;28:567-575.
3. Nepomuceno RL, Boxer Wachler BS, Kim JM, Scruggs R, Sato M. Laser in situ keratomileusis for hyperopia with the LADARVision 4000 with centration on the coaxially sighted corneal light reflex. *J Cataract Refract Surg.* 2004;30:1281-1286.
4. Okamoto S, Kimura K, Funakura M, Ikeda N, Hiramatsu H, Bains HS. Comparison of wavefront-guided aspheric laser in situ keratomileusis for myopia: Coaxially sighted corneal-light-reflex versus line-of-sight centration. *J Cataract Refract Surg.* 2011;37:1951-1960.

Some portions of the text reprinted with permission from Arba Mosquera S, Ewering T. New asymmetric centration strategy combining pupil and corneal vertex information for ablation procedures in refractive surgery: Theoretical background. *J Refract Surg.* 2012;28:567-575.

10
QUESTION

How Do I Manage Suction Loss During LASIK?

Pravin Krishna Vaddavalli, MD and Vardhaman P. Kankariya, MD

LASIK has become the most frequently performed corneal refractive surgery, and creation of the flap is arguably the most important step. The flap may be created with the microkeratome, or more recently with femtosecond laser technology. Although femtosecond lasers provide better uniformity and predictability of dimensions to the LASIK flap, complications such as suction loss still do occur with both of the flap makers. During the creation of the flap, the suction ring may lose suction for a variety of reasons, and the applanation plate may become separated from the cornea, creating a partial flap. The reported incidence varies between 0.06% to 4% of eyes undergoing LASIK.[1]

Suction loss during flap creation can be attributed to a number of patient-related factors, such as anxiety leading to lid squeezing; head and eye movements; anatomical factors like small palpebral fissure, deep set eyes, prominent brow ridge; and rarely, defective suction apparatus, conjunctival chemosis, and epithelial breakthrough. Apart from these causes, flat corneal curvature is a risk factor unique to the mechanical microkeratome. The risk of suction loss is reportedly decreasing with advancement in femtosecond laser platforms, leading to an increase in the pulse frequency and a reduction in duration of the procedure itself.

Consequences and management of the suction loss during a femtosecond laser-assisted LASIK depend on the stage at which it was encountered. If it occurs before starting the laser lamellar cut, a suction ring is reapplied and the procedure is completed normally. On the contrary, if the suction is lost after partial propagation of laser, an incomplete/partial flap is encountered. In this situation, the same suction ring is immediately reapplied using conjunctival markings as the reference mark, docked with same patient interface (applanation cone), and a second pass is made at the same depth and utilizing identical settings for flap diameter, but without the pocket creation (with "pocket off" setting). The excellent accuracy and reproducibility of femtosecond laser is utilized

Henderson BA, Yoo SH. *Curbside Consultation in Refractive and Lens-Based Surgery: 49 Clinical Questions* (pp 37-39)
© 2015 SLACK Incorporated

during the second pass and the flap is usually created at the same plane. It is important to note that the same patient interface (applanation cone) should be used because each cone is calibrated and different cones may have slight differences in plate thickness, which may result in the creation of two interfaces.

Furthermore, if suction is lost during the side cut, the diameter of the side cut is decreased by 0.5 or 1 mm. The suction ring is reapplied in exactly the same position and only the side cut function is performed just inside the outside diameter of the lamellar cut. It is critical that the centration is optimally maintained while docking. In such situations, the integration of real-time optical coherence tomography (OCT) with femtosecond laser technology may improve precision for side cut creation.

Even with all these precautions, crossing of the two cut planes may occur because of differences in applanation pressure, hydration conditions, and chemosis. Therefore, in the case of a double pass, some surgeons recommend dissecting the LASIK flap from the opposite side of the hinge (vs the conventional dissection from the hinge side). This may help avoid false passage. After ablation with the excimer laser, these step or line types of stromal regularities are diminished. In the largest series by Tomita et al involving 71 eyes of 70 patients with suction loss during femtosecond laser-enabled LASIK, all eyes had good results.[2] A recent study from Munoz et al compared the results of LASIK with an uneventful single femtosecond laser pass with that of a double pass that was performed for retreatment of the pupillary area involving partial flap.[3] Visual acuity, refractive outcomes, and anterior corneal higher-order aberrations were comparable between eyes. An additional femtosecond laser pass performed immediately after an incomplete flap due to intraoperative suction loss provided good visual and optical outcomes.

If the surgeon is uncomfortable with a second pass, photorefractive keratectomy (PRK) with adjuvant mitomycin C (MMC) can be a good option. It is advisable to wait 1 month before attempting PRK in order to note refractive stability. Smajda et al demonstrated that the stromal step corresponding to the area where the suction was lost diminished in intensity after excimer ablation, and corneal epithelium compensated for stromal abnormalities and provided good visual results.[4] Use of MMC to decrease the risk of haze formation cannot be overstated, and we recommend using MMC longer (30 seconds to 1 minute) than the conventional 12 to 15 seconds. In the case of suction loss with mechanical microkeratome, we advise a similar approach of PRK with MMC after a period of 1 month of stability. We do not advocate a double pass with the microkeratome due to its suboptimal reproducibility in achieved flap thickness, which may lead to sight-threatening complications.

There are certain recommendations to decrease risk of suction loss during flap creation. Preoperative counseling to alleviate anxiety helps to improve patient cooperation during the procedure because noncooperation and eye or head movements are the most common causes of the suction loss. Recognition of anatomical risk factors implicated in occurrence of suction loss, such as tight orbits and small palpebral fissure, during preoperative assessment, inspection of the suction apparatus, and vigilance during the procedure may decrease incidence of suction loss as well. With the growing experience of surgeons and advancements in technology, incidence of suction loss may further decline, improving the overall safety of the most common elective procedure on the human body.

References

1. Haft P, Yoo SH, Kymionis GD, Ide T, O'Brien TP, Culbertson WW. Complications of LASIK flaps made by the IntraLase 15- and 30-kHz femtosecond lasers. *J Refract Surg*. 2009;25:979-984.
2. Tomita M, Watabe M, Nakamura T, Nakamura N, Tsuru T, Waring GO IV. Management and outcomes of suction loss during LASIK flap creation with a femtosecond laser. *J Refract Surg*. 2012;28:32-36.

3. Muñoz G, Albarrán-Diego C, Ferrer-Blasco T, Javaloy J, García-Lázaro S. Single versus double femtosecond laser pass for incomplete laser in situ keratomileusis flap in contralateral eyes: Visual and optical outcomes. *J Cataract Refract Surg.* 2012;38:8-15.

4. Smadja D, Santhiago MR, Mello GR, Espana EM, Krueger RR. Suction loss during thin-flap femto-LASIK: Management and beneficial refractive effect of the epithelium. *J Cataract Refract Surg.* 2012;38:902-905.

WHAT SHOULD I DO IF MY PATIENT HAS A DECENTERED FLAP?

George D. Kymionis, MD, PhD and George A. Kontadakis, MD, MSc

Flap decentration is an uncommon complication of conventional LASIK with mechanical microkeratome and has been practically eliminated with femtosecond lasers.[1] When it occurs, however, flap decentration can undermine LASIK results. A significantly decentered flap whose edge lies within the optical ablation zone can induce astigmatism and visually disabling higher-order aberrations.[2] Surgeons should therefore be very meticulous in the placement of the microkeratome in order to reduce the risk of this complication.

In our practice, in order to avoid decentration when using a mechanical microkeratome, we carefully place the suction ring in a well-centered position symmetrical to anatomic landmarks such as the pupil and limbus. In hyperopic patients, where there may be a large angle kappa, the flap should be centered relative to the visual axis rather than the pupil. High astigmatism and short white-to-white measurements are associated with higher risk for decentered flaps. Eye drift after suction engagement may dislocate a properly aligned suction ring and can be managed with gentle displacement of the ring in the opposite direction.[2] Another significant variable is patient cooperation. An uncooperative patient is more likely to end up with a poorly centered suction and a decentered flap.

With the use of femtosecond lasers, after applying the suction ring and docking the laser cone, the opportunity remains to adjust the flap placement on the cornea while viewing the patient's pupil. Thus, in our experience, significant flap decentration is very unlikely.

If the flap is decentered, our approach depends largely on the extent of decentration and the diameter of the optical zone that we intend to treat. In hyperopic, astigmatic, and wavefront-guided corrections, the treatment zone is usually larger. If a well-centered ablation zone lies within the limits of the misaligned flap, we can proceed with the excimer laser ablation without any concerns. When the limit of the flap is inside the ablation zone, we first check whether we can

Henderson BA, Yoo SH. *Curbside Consultation in Refractive and Lens-Based Surgery: 49 Clinical Questions* (pp 41-42)
© 2015 SLACK Incorporated

reduce the treatment zone to be inside the limits of the flap without compromising the result of the operation. Considerations such as pupil diameter and eye dominance are taken into account. In both cases, the measurement and calibration of the laser treatment are better done before lifting the flap, to avoid unnecessary manipulations if the operation must be postponed. Other surgeons suggest measuring the dimensions of the stromal bed with a caliper after lifting the flap to obtain a more accurate estimation of the ablation zone and flap limit.[3] In the case of femtosecond lasers, avoiding lifting a decentered flap is very important because, if left intact, the tissue can later be treated by the surgeon as if the flap had not been created at all.

If the ablation zone cannot fit inside the limits of the decentered flap, then the procedure must be aborted. In cases of mechanical microkeratome flaps, I prefer to wait a few months before reoperating. Usually, 3 to 6 months is sufficient to allow the patient's topography and refraction to completely stabilize and the tissue to be as compact as possible, such that the flap remains in place. At reoperation, I prefer to create a deeper flap (20 to 60 μm deeper) in order to avoid coincidence of the new cut with the previous one,[4] then continue the procedure as initially planned. In cases of flaps created with a femtosecond laser, if the flap was lifted during the first procedure, my steps are similar as previously described for the mechanical microkeratome. If the flap was not lifted, the tissue can be treated as if no flap had been created and the laser parameters can be set as in the first procedure.

When tissue thickness is insufficient to create a deeper flap, a preferable treatment option is photorefractive keratectomy with adjuvant application of mitomycin C.[5] A no-touch transepithelial photorefractive keratectomy can also be performed. Flap decentration is not one of the most feared complications of LASIK because, if properly treated, the final visual outcome is not compromised. Furthermore, meticulous placement of the microkeratome significantly reduces the chances of this occurring.

References

1. Moshirfar M, Gardiner JP, Schliesser JA, et al. Laser in situ keratomileusis flap complications using mechanical microkeratomes versus femtosecond laser: Retrospective comparison. *J Cataract Refract Surg.* 2010;36:1925-1933.
2. Schallhorn SC, Amesbury EC, Tanzer DJ. Avoidance, recognition, and management of LASIK complications. *Am J Ophthalmol.* 2006;141(4):733-739.
3. Cummings A, Lavery F. Flap complications. In: Agarwal A, Agarwal A, Jacob S, eds. *Refractive Surgery.* 2nd ed. New Delhi, India: Jaypee Brothers Ltd; 2009:411-418.
4. Tekwani NH, Chalita MR, Krueger RR. Secondary microkeratome-induced flap interference with the pathway of the primary flap. *Ophthalmology.* 2003;110(7):1379-1383.
5. Kymionis GD, Portaliou DM, Karavitaki AE, et al. LASIK flap buttonhole treated immediately by PRK with mitomycin C. *J Refract Surg.* 2010;26(3):225-228.

12

HOW DO I MANAGE A BUTTONHOLE OR FREE CAP DURING LASIK?

Lingmin He, MD, MS and Edward E. Manche, MD

A buttonhole defect or free corneal cap complicates 0.2% to 2.6% of primary LASIK surgeries,[1] but proper diagnosis and appropriate management often lead to satisfactory postoperative outcomes.

Free caps are most commonly seen when flat corneas (< 40 diopters [D]) are cut with mechanical keratomes and are rarely seen when using femtosecond lasers. In most of these cases, LASIK surgery can be completed without further complications. It is important to properly align the flap in the correct position with the help of peripheral corneal markings and place a bandage contact lens overnight to help prevent loss of the cap. Misalignment of the flap may lead to complications such as induced astigmatism, flap striae, and epithelial ingrowth.

Buttonhole flap defects usually occur when the microkeratome blade does not maintain a consistent cutting plane throughout the cornea, but prematurely cleaves the epithelium and leaves a portion of the flap uncut. Risk factors for this complication include steep corneas (likely because the corneal tissue buckles posteriorly), previous corneal scarring, blade defects, and use of the same blade to cut the second eye. Increased use of femtosecond lasers to create the LASIK flap has reduced but not eliminated this complication. Vertical gas breakthrough (VGB) into the epithelium can occur due to a previous break in Bowman's layer. The interface gas moves through the defect, causing an area of stroma to avoid photodisruption by the femtosecond laser. While not a true buttonhole, VGB can result in a tear or hole in the flap if the surgeon attempts to elevate the flap.

When buttonholes develop, they can result in extensive epithelial ingrowth around the edges of the defect, which may lead to significant visual distortion by creating irregular astigmatism, flap necrosis, and scarring (Figure 12-1). Thus, it remains an important entity to recognize. Appropriate management can lead to optimal visual outcomes even in difficult cases with extensive central epithelial ingrowth.

Henderson BA, Yoo SH. *Curbside Consultation in Refractive and Lens-Based Surgery: 49 Clinical Questions* (pp 43-45)
© 2015 SLACK Incorporated

Figure 12-1. (A) Central buttonhole defect with extensive epithelial ingrowth and macrostriae with a superior island of epithelial ingrowth near the flap hinge. (B) Topography of the same eye shows central flattening with significant distortion in the areas of the epithelial ingrowth.

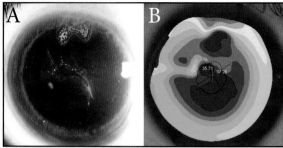

It is critical to recognize the presence of a buttonhole during the initial surgery. If a buttonhole is noted during creation of the flap, the best course of action is to abort the surgery. Continuation with the excimer laser treatment may result in poor adhesion at the flap interface that can lead to epithelial ingrowth, scarring, irregular astigmatism, and ultimately loss of visual acuity. In our experience, if the flap is repositioned with good alignment relative to the stromal bed and no excimer laser ablation is performed, most significant complications of buttonholes can be avoided.

We generally prescribe topical steroids 4 times a day for the first week, then taper based on the presence of any corneal haze or fibrosis. We review patients on postoperative day 1; weeks 1, 2, and 3; and months 1 and 3. Other groups have suggested hourly steroids for the first 2 to 3 days to minimize the risk of diffuse lamellar keratitis.[2] Early retreatment can lead to refractive surprises as wound remodeling occurs and to flap interface complications due to the lack of a tight barrier to epithelial ingrowth.

We feel that retreatments should be attempted only after several months in order to ensure that the epithelium is smooth, the refraction has stabilized, and subepithelial scarring is no longer progressing. When retreatment appears safe, we prefer transepithelial phototherapeutic keratectomy (PTK) (50 μm) with photorefractive keratectomy (PRK) and adjuvant mitomycin C (MMC). We perform transepithelial PTK using a "no-touch" technique, followed immediately by PRK with MMC. It is important to avoid mechanical manipulation of the flap so that its edges are not dislodged or disrupted. Other techniques include alcohol-assisted removal of the epithelium followed by PRK treatment with MMC. We do not recommend recutting or relifting the flap because this can lead to poor tissue adherence at the edges and other serious complications.[3]

In cases where flap defects are associated with extensive epithelial ingrowth, we suggest lifting the flap and mechanically scraping the epithelial ingrowth. Unfortunately, the reported recurrence rates after removal of epithelial ingrowth are as high as 44%. One technique to reduce the recurrence of ingrowth is to create a tight seal at the epithelial interface with sutures.[4] However, we have recently begun applying fibrin glue around the edges of the LASIK flap and the area of the buttonhole to the same effect. The advantage of this technique is that the glues are dissolvable, induce less astigmatism, and can be used even when the defect is central. The patients we have treated so far have avoided flap amputation and have good visual outcomes, despite having extensive topographic irregularities present on initial examination.[5]

Buttonhole creation during LASIK surgery can lead to significant visual impairment if it is not recognized and epithelial ingrowth develops. If treatment is aborted, however, patients can usually be monitored with tight adherence at the flap and buttonhole edges. Even when epithelial ingrowth does develop or there is poor tissue apposition, new treatments can lead to good final visual results.

References

1. Leung AT, Rao SK, Cheng AC, Yu EW, Fan DS, Lam DS. Pathogenesis and management of laser in situ keratomileusis flap buttonhole. *J Cataract Refract Surg*. 2000;26:358-362.
2. Harissi-Dagher M, Todani A, Melki SA. Laser in situ keratomileusis buttonhole: Classification and management algorithm. *J Cataract Refract Surg*. 2008;34:1892-1899.
3. Rubinfeld RS, Hardten DR, Donnenfeld ED, et al. To lift or recut: Changing trends in LASIK enhancement. *J Cataract Refract Surg*. 2003;29:2306-2317.
4. Rojas MC, Lumba JD, Manche EE. Treatment of epithelial ingrowth after laser in situ keratomileusis with mechanical debridement and flap suturing. *Arch Ophthalmol*. 2004;122:997-1001.
5. He L, Manche EE. Fibrin glue for prevention of recurrent epithelial ingrowth under a LASIK flap with a central buttonhole defect. *J Cataract Refract Surg*. 2012;38:1857-1860.

SHOULD I USE MITOMYCIN C WITH ALL OF MY PRK CASES?

Vasilios F. Diakonis, MD, PhD and Vardhaman P. Kankariya, MD

In 2001, 9 years after experimental studies of rabbit corneas, the first clinical trial of photorefractive keratectomy (PRK) with adjuvant mitomycin C (MMC) by Majmudar et al demonstrated satisfactory refractive outcomes by modulating corneal healing response and controlling haze formation.[1] MMC is a chemotherapeutic antibiotic agent that exerts its action by crosslinking cellular DNA, thus inhibiting mitosis and m-RNA synthesis and ultimately leading to cellular apoptosis, most powerfully in fibroblasts and vascular endothelial cells. In refractive surgery, MMC is used for its cytostatic effect on keratocytes, preventing their replication, activation, and production of new collagen to modulate corneal wound healing and haze formation after PRK.

The first off-label protocol described a 2-minute 0.02% MMC exposure on the bare corneal stroma after photoablation, followed by meticulous rinsing of the cornea with 20 cc of balanced saline solution (BSS). Due to concerns regarding MMC's long-term safety and adverse effects on ocular tissues, the protocol has changed and suggestions have been proposed to reduce exposure time and concentration. Although a standardized nomogram for MMC's intraoperative use has yet to be established, most surgeons have linked the exposure time of MMC on the attempted correction (low corrections = short exposure, high corrections = longer exposure) on their experience and outcomes. On the other hand, there seems to be a consensus on the MMC concentration because most surgeons use 0.02%.

Today, prophylactic MMC in PRK typically does not exceed 30 seconds for high attempted corrections (–5 to –10 diopters [D]) and 15 seconds for low attempted corrections (–1 to –4 D). Two minutes of exposure is now reserved for complicated cases such as haze and retreatments. Nevertheless, there are still concerns about possible toxic effects, especially on the endothelial cell layer. A few reports reveal decreased endothelial cell density,[2] while the majority of authors report

Henderson BA, Yoo SH. *Curbside Consultation in Refractive
and Lens-Based Surgery: 49 Clinical Questions* (pp 47-48)
© 2015 SLACK Incorporated

no endothelial cell loss.[3] This drawback deters many surgeons from using MMC in all PRK cases, and most choose to use it only in higher attempted corrections where risk of haze is greatest.

The ultimate goal of MMC in surface ablations is to eliminate haze formation and further optimize refractive and visual outcomes. Known risk factors for haze formation include high ametropias as well as age, sex, and sun exposure; thus, no patient is inherently protected. All things considered, the principle of "all or none" may apply to prophylactic MMC use in refractive surgery. In our opinion, all PRK patients should receive MMC intraoperatively in order to reduce the risk of haze. Even though most corneas undergoing PRK will not develop haze, the use of MMC targets those few that otherwise would.

Conclusion

Refractive surgery is an elective procedure, and perfection in terms of outcomes is required for all patients. MMC is a useful tool for refractive surgeons to eliminate troubling complications that may lead to visual impairment. We use MMC in all surface ablations. We apply MMC for 15 seconds on corrections up to –5 D and for 30 seconds above –5 D. Long-term follow-up studies (over 5 years) are necessary to abolish concerns about possible toxic effects, especially on the endothelial cell layer.

References

1. Majmudar PA, Forstot SL, Nirankari VS, et al. Topical Mitomycin-C for subepithelial fibrosis after corneal surgery. *Ophthalmology.* 2000;107:89-94.
2. Morales AJ, Zadok D, Mora-Retana R, Martinez-Gama E, Robledo NE, Chayet AS. Intraoperative mitomycin and corneal endothelium after photorefractive keratectomy. *Am J Ophthalmol.* 2006;142:400-404.
3. Diakonis VF, Pallikaris A, Kymionis GD, Markomanolakis MM. Alterations in endothelial cell density after photorefractive keratectomy with adjuvant mitomycin. *Am J Ophthalmol.* 2007;144(1):99-103.

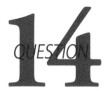

WHAT SHOULD I DO ABOUT A LARGE EPITHELIAL DEFECT THAT OCCURS DURING LASIK?

Vardhaman P. Kankariya, MD and Vasilios F. Diakonis, MD, PhD

Epithelial defects are among the most common intraoperative complications of primary LASIK cases, with an estimated incidence of 1.6% to 5%. Although most are peripheral, small, and innocuous, central and large defects also occur, predisposing the eye toward more concerning postoperative complications. In these cases, patients may experience increased discomfort and delayed visual recovery, as well as increased risk of developing diffuse lamellar keratitis (DLK). Other complications include recurrent epithelial erosion, epithelial ingrowth, undercorrection, and microbial keratitis.[1]

Optimizing management by understanding risk factors, minimizing intraoperative epithelial damage, and employing careful intra- and postoperative management should reduce the incidence of these defects and improve outcomes of LASIK.

Understanding Risk Factors

Inadvertent minor trauma by forceps, spatula, or a cannula tip can lead to small intraoperative epithelial defects. Larger defects, on the other hand, typically occur in eyes that are anatomically predisposed to corneal epithelial sloughing. Risk factors include epithelial basement membrane dystrophy (EBMD), older age, thicker cornea, severe dry eye, and diabetes mellitus (due to pathologic changes in junctional complexes).

Microkeratomes may contribute to the formation of epithelial defects by creating frictional forces across the cornea during excursion. The attributable risk varies by brand and type, with angular motion microkeratomes implicated more than transverse.

Henderson BA, Yoo SH. *Curbside Consultation in Refractive and Lens-Based Surgery: 49 Clinical Questions* (pp 49-51)
© 2015 SLACK Incorporated

Iatrogenic causes include excessive anesthesia leading to junctional complex damage at the epithelial basement membrane and corneal desiccation from prolonged exposure.[2]

Minimizing Risk of Intraoperative Epithelial Defects

Femtosecond laser microkeratomes produce smaller shearing forces and fewer epithelial defects than do mechanical microkeratomes.[3] Careful screening with exclusion of high-risk patients, along with adoption of epithelium-friendly surgical protocol in routine LASIK, will minimize the risk associated with mechanical microkeratomes.

Patients should be carefully screened for any history of recurrent erosions, dry eye, or signs of EBMD. Older patients and those with diabetes or thicker corneas should be thoroughly evaluated and counseled regarding the risk of this complication. If the corneal epithelium is loose, advanced surface ablation procedures are preferable. A microsponge applicator can be used to test for loose epithelium in suspicious cases.

In all routine LASIK procedures, preoperative anesthetics must be used judiciously to prevent disruption of corneal epithelial adhesion complexes. I prefer generous lubrication of the corneal surface with balanced saline solution (BSS) before use of the microkeratome to reduce frictional force at the time of flap cut. Others have advocated releasing the suction ring vacuum as the microkeratome is withdrawn. Careful execution of each step of the procedure will minimize the risk of epithelial damage.

Intraoperative- and Postoperative Management of Large Epithelial Defects

The surgeon should inspect the corneal flap, noting the presence and extent of any epithelial defects and taking care to avoid further damage in subsequent steps. With gentle handling of the flap, it is usually safe to proceed with ablation. After ablation, the flap should be returned to its original position carefully because flap edges adjacent to epithelium that is sloughing due to edema may encourage epithelial ingrowth. Torn edges of epithelium may be debrided with a Beaver blade (Beaver-Visitec International, Inc) to encourage epithelialization.

A bandage soft contact lens stabilizes the epithelial sheet and promotes healing. It is kept in place until the epithelium is completely healed—several days in cases of large defects. Frequent postoperative examinations should be conducted to assess epithelial healing and to identify and manage possible complications, such as epithelial ingrowth, diffuse lamellar keratitis, and recurrent corneal erosion. Other elements of complete follow-up care include an adequate course of broad-spectrum antibiotics to prevent corneal infection, frequent steroids for prophylaxis and treatment of DLK, and preservative-free lubricants. Continuing lubrication beyond resolution of the epithelial defect serves to support the corneal surface and to allow the hemidesmosomal attachments to form.[4]

Finally, in the event of an intraoperative epithelial defect in the first eye, the fellow eye procedure should be undertaken only after discussion with the patient. The fellow eye must be examined on high magnification under slit-lamp (oblique and retro-illumination) for subtle signs of EBMD. Recognizing the limited sensitivity of this technique (5% of eyes with EBMD appear normal on slit-lamp exam) and that advanced surface ablation reduces recurrent epithelial erosions in the patients, we prefer to use advanced surface ablation on the fellow eye even in the absence of signs of EBMD.

References

1. Tekwani NH, Huang D. Risk factors for intraoperative epithelial defect in laser in-situ keratomileusis. *Am J Ophthalmol.* 2002;134:311-316.
2. Randleman JB, Lynn MJ, Banning CS, Stulting RD. Risk factors for epithelial defect formation during laser in situ keratomileusis. *J Cataract Refract Surg.* 2007;33(10):1738-1743.
3. Kymionis GD, Kankariya VP, Plaka AD, Reinstein DZ. Femtosecond laser technology in corneal refractive surgery: A review. *J Refract Surg.* 2012;28(12):912-920.
4. Smirennaia E, Sheludchenko V, Kourenkova N, Kashnikova O. Management of corneal epithelial defects following laser in situ keratomileusis. *J Refract Surg.* 2001;17:S196-S199.

SECTION III

POSTOPERATIVE COMPLICATIONS

15

HOW DO I MANAGE DIFFUSE LAMELLAR KERATITIS AFTER LASIK? HOW DOES THIS DIFFER FROM PRESSURE-INDUCED INTERLAMELLAR STROMAL KERATITIS?

Matthew J. Weiss, MD and Sonia H. Yoo, MD

The introduction of corneal flaps, as in LASIK, has led to a unique alteration of corneal anatomy associated with its own category of postoperative complications. Specifically, the interface created by the lamellar dissection of the corneal stroma during this keratorefractive procedure represents a potential space that can become the site of inflammatory cells or fluid accumulation. Diffuse lamellar keratitis (DLK) is a noninfectious inflammatory condition affecting this interface. Pressure-induced interlamellar stromal keratitis (PISK) is a diffuse haze related to interlamellar fluid accumulation involving the interface. Although the etiologies for these two conditions are distinct, they can appear very similar clinically. Because the treatment for DLK involves frequent topical steroids that can actually exacerbate the condition of a patient with PISK, early differentiation and implementation of appropriate treatment measures are critical to achieving a favorable outcome.

DLK is one of the more common complications among LASIK patients, with an incidence likely less than 3% (reports range from 0.13% to 18.9%).[1] The condition is defined by a sterile infiltrate of white blood cells at the level of the interface. Confocal microscopy examination reveals primarily mononuclear cells and granulocytes.[2] Although various exogenous and endogenous factors appear to contribute to the development of DLK, bacterial endotoxins are among the most important.[1] Endotoxin-related cases of DLK typically result from contaminated sterilizing systems and can yield epidemics. Chemicals, cleaners, and equipment commonly used in refractive suites have also been implicated in the onset of DLK.[1] Therefore, we recommend monitoring for outbreaks so that they can be addressed promptly. Other risk factors for the development of DLK include patient conditions such as dry eye, anterior basement membrane dystrophies, atopic and autoimmune diseases, and staphylococcal marginal keratitis. In order to minimize the risk

Henderson BA, Yoo SH. *Curbside Consultation in Refractive and Lens-Based Surgery: 49 Clinical Questions* (pp 55-56)
© 2015 SLACK Incorporated

of DLK, we suggest addressing any ocular surface comorbidities prior to performing refractive surgery.

Because prompt treatment is vital to the patient's prognosis, DLK must be diagnosed rapidly and accurately.[1] DLK typically presents in the immediate postoperative period, generally 1 to 5 days after surgery. A typical patient presents with foreign body sensation, no significant pain, no conjunctival injection, normal intraocular pressure, and minimal change in vision. These signs and symptoms are important to identify because they can help distinguish DLK from other conditions such as PISK and infectious processes.[3] DLK appears as a peripheral granular interface infiltrate that progresses over time to a diffuse dense haze with scarring in 4 classic stages, as described by Linebarger et al.[3] In stage 1, DLK has only a peripheral granular infiltration. In stage 2, the infiltration extends to involve the paracentral cornea. By stage 3, the central cornea and visual axis are affected and the lamellar infiltrate becomes denser. Finally, in stage 4, the infiltrate consolidates and causes dense haze, scarring, and flap necrosis.[3] The ability to distinguish these stages clinically is vital because the appearance dictates the necessary treatment.

DLK is highly steroid responsive, therefore topical and/or oral steroids are the primary mode of treatment.[3] In stage 1 DLK, we recommend initiating treatment with frequent administration of topical steroids. If the inflammation has progressed to stage 2 or beyond, oral steroids are generally indicated in addition to drops. As an adjunct to steroid therapy, one can consider lifting the flap and irrigating the LASIK interface. Although this technique is usually performed in unresponsive stage 2 and all stage 3 disease, flap lifting in stage 4 should be approached with extreme caution because it can lead to irreversible damage of friable and necrotic tissue.[3]

In contrast to DLK, PISK is a very rare complication related to elevated intraocular pressure in LASIK. The incidence of PISK is not known because there are only a few published reports of the process.[4] In this condition, postoperative steroid use leads to an acute rise in intraocular pressure, which in turn yields a diffuse haze at the level of the LASIK interface. The interface haze of PISK is highly visually significant, appears more reticular than the haze of DLK, and can be associated with a fluid cleft. Anterior segment optical coherence tomography (OCT) is useful in defining the presence of this kind of fluid accumulation.[4] Because this process is secondary to a steroid response, the onset is much later than in DLK; typically, these patients present 1 to 3 weeks postoperatively.[3] For this reason, we recommend routine monitoring of intraocular pressure. Notably, if a fluid cleft is present, the measured pressure can be falsely low. Therefore, if you suspect PISK, we advise checking intraocular pressure from a peripheral location with a Tono-Pen (Reichert Inc.) or Schiøtz tonometer, which is less prone to measurement error in these patients.[2]

Elevated intraocular pressure and delays in diagnosis put these patients at risk of developing glaucomatous optic neuropathies with resultant visual field loss.[2] Therefore, early diagnosis and treatment are vital. When PISK is diagnosed, steroids must be tapered and stopped as soon as possible, and pressure-lowering medications should be started. On the correct treatment, vision can improve within hours.[4] Patients should be monitored on treatment until intraocular pressure normalizes and any interface fluid resolves. With prompt and appropriate management, PISK is associated with a good visual prognosis.[3]

References

1. Gritz DC. LASIK interface keratitis: epidemiology, diagnosis and care. *Curr Opin Ophthalmol.* 2011;22:251-255.
2. Tourtas T, Kopsachilis N, Meiller R, Kruse FE, Cursiefen C. Pressure-induced interlamellar stromal keratitis after laser in situ keratomileusis. *Cornea.* 2011;30(8):920-923.
3. Linebarger EJ, Hardten DR, Lindstrom RL. Diffuse lamellar keratitis: diagnosis and management. *J Cataract Refract Surg.* 2000;26(7):1072-1077.
4. Levinger E, Slomovic A, Bahar I, Slomovic AR. Diagnosis of steroid-induced elevated intraocular pressure and associated lamellar keratitis after laser in situ keratomileusis using optical coherence tomography. *J Cataract Refract Surg.* 2009;35:386-388.

16

WHAT SHOULD I DO IN CASE OF LASIK FLAP DISLOCATION?

Majid Moshirfar, MD and Jason N. Edmonds, MD

Flap dislocation is a rare but feared complication of LASIK surgery. A careful, stepwise approach allows the ophthalmologist to adequately address this issue, prevent complications, and preserve visual acuity.

Timing of flap dislocation is important. Your first consideration in addressing a patient with a LASIK flap dislocation is to identify the timing of dislocation in the postoperative course. Flap dislocations in the first 48 to 72 hours are most often due to poor adhesion. Risk factors include heavy blinking or squeezing of the eyelids, severe dry eye, and side-cut retraction. Use of intraoperative brimonidine has been shown to cause flap slippage, increasing the risk of dislocation. Late flap dislocation is most often due to trauma, often from fingers, tools, airbag deployment, animals, tree branches, and balls used in recreational activities.[1] Flap dislocations have been reported as late as 13 years after surgery.

The severity of the flap dislocation also guides the type and timing of intervention. Minor flap dislocations may present with subtle clinical findings such as macrostriae or flap folds (Figure 16-1). Severe flap dislocations may cause near-complete to complete flap dehiscence. Dislocations involving the central flap may lead to more or worse sequelae than those limited to the periphery.

Careful examination at the slit-lamp is one of the most important steps in managing flap dislocation. Any epithelial ingrowth must be recognized. Complications of epithelial ingrowth include focal flap elevation at the edge or centrally, extension into the visual axis that compromises vision, and, rarely, flap melt, especially if epithelial ingrowth is not swiftly addressed. Epithelial ingrowth can induce irregular astigmatism and hyperopia. Identifying and addressing epithelial ingrowth at initial surgical intervention can reverse these complications and optimize postoperative outcomes.

Henderson BA, Yoo SH. *Curbside Consultation in Refractive and Lens-Based Surgery: 49 Clinical Questions* (pp 57-59)
© 2015 SLACK Incorporated

Figure 16-1. Macrostriae in the LASIK flap following traumatic dislocation.

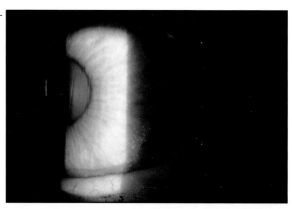

Figure 16-2. Epithelial ingrowth beneath the LASIK flap following traumatic flap dislocation.

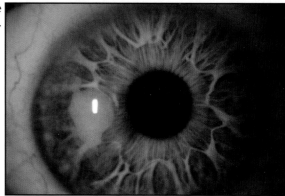

The management of early flap dislocation is relatively straightforward. Early dislocation should be addressed at the laser microscope, where the flap can be refloated with the irrigation cannula. Because epithelial injury can increase the risk of developing diffuse lamellar keratitis (DLK), careful inspection should be performed and a bandage contact lens applied if any such injury is identified. After flap replacement, we recommend treatment with a fourth-generation fluoroquinolone and topical steroid. Maintain close follow-up to monitor for DLK and epithelial ingrowth.

The management of late flap dislocation is dictated by severity. Some minor dislocations involving the peripheral flap and causing folds or striae with preservation of uncorrected visual acuity can be treated medically. Look carefully with the slit-lamp microscope for epithelial ingrowth and defects. In the case of flap folds or striae, we recommend treatment with a topical fluoroquinolone and topical steroid. For epithelial injury, we recommend placement of a bandage contact lens. These patients should be closely monitored for the development of DLK and epithelial ingrowth (Figure 16-2). Mild dislocations with poor visual acuity may require surgical intervention, including repositioning the flap with Weck-Cel (Beaver-Visitec International, Inc) sponges or the irrigation cannula.

Severe dislocations resulting in partial or full flap dehiscence can pose the greatest challenge to refractive surgeons. Potential complications include infection, epithelial ingrowth, or even complete epithelialization of the exposed stroma. Epithelial ingrowth must be addressed immediately. Considering the manipulations this entails, we recommend proceeding to the operating room and administering a lid block when necessary. Remove all epithelium from the flap interface and stroma. You may need to lift the flap to access areas of ingrowth that are not already exposed. We reposition the flap using an irrigating cannula and Weck-Cel sponges. We then place multiple

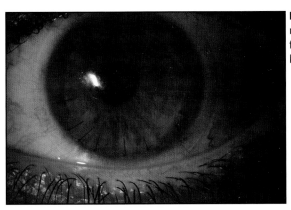

Figure 16-3. Multiple simple interrupted 10-0 nylon sutures with knots rotated away from the flap (but not buried) with a bandage contact lens.

radially oriented simple 10-0 nylon interrupted sutures along with fibrin glue to keep the flap in place and reduce the risk of future epithelial ingrowth. To minimize stress on the flap, we do not bury the knots; instead, we rotate them away from the flap (Figure 16-3).[2] Fibrin glue seals the flap edges, and a bandage contact lens is placed.[3] Close follow-up is essential. We recommend stepwise removal of the sutures starting 2 weeks postoperatively, maintaining a topical fluoroquinolone and topical steroid while sutures are present.

Appropriate management of flap dislocation depends on the timing, severity, and sequelae, such as DLK and epithelial ingrowth. A meticulous approach and attention to detail can minimize complications and preserve visual acuity.

References

1. Kim HJ, Silverman CM. Traumatic dislocation of flaps 4 and 9 years after surgery. *J Refract Surg.* 2010;26(6):447-452.
2. Moshirfar M, Anderson E, Taylor N, Hsu M. Management of a traumatic flap dislocation seven years after LASIK. *Case Rep Ophthlamol Med.* 2011;2011:514780.
3. Anderson NJ, Hardten DR. Fibrin glue for the prevention of epithelial ingrowth after laser in situ keratomileusis. *J Cataract Refract Surg.* 2003;29:1425-1429.

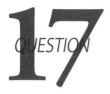

QUESTION

17

When Should I Perform a Second Procedure in Patients With Flap Striae?

Jordon G. Lubahn, MD and William W. Culbertson, MD

Flap striae are a frustrating and sometimes significant complication after LASIK. Fortunately, most cases of striae are not visually significant, especially if outside the visual axis. However, the reported incidence of visually significant striae requiring management is almost 2%.[1]

Striae are best observed at the slit-lamp, which is easiest after dilation (Figure 17-1), but can also be highlighted with fluorescein staining of the cornea. Typically, the folds are in the direction of the hinge—horizontally with a nasal hinge and vertically with a superior hinge. The exam findings range from fine parallel lines in the periphery of the flap, to extension of fine lines or a "basket weave" pattern into the visual axis, to large, dense folds throughout the entire flap.[2]

These abnormalities can cause decreased vision, monocular diplopia, glare, and induced astigmatism, all of which can be neutralized with a hard contact lens. Significance of striae can also be assessed using the "Maddox rod effect," wherein the patient draws a sketch of the appearance of a bright light source with specific attention to the orientation of the starburst light rays; similar to the line seen in Maddox rod testing, the direction of starburst will be perpendicular to the flap striae.[3]

Striae in the tissue are thought to emanate from misalignment of the corneal flap after flap replacement, movement of the corneal flap during the first postoperative day, and the tenting effect of the corneal flap over the ablated stromal bed.[2]

Risk factors for this complication include a small hinge, thin flap, large myopic correction, overhydration with excessive stroking of the flap, and use of topical vasoconstricting agents (eg, brimonidine, phenylephrine).

Although sometimes difficult to detect after surgery given other postoperative corneal changes, these defects can be seen immediately after LASIK is performed when examining the patient at the slit-lamp before discharge. If not seen initially, significant striae should be seen on exam on

Henderson BA, Yoo SH. *Curbside Consultation in Refractive and Lens-Based Surgery: 49 Clinical Questions* (pp 61-63)
© 2015 SLACK Incorporated

Figure 17-1. Examples from separate eyes of fine, central flap striae after LASIK.

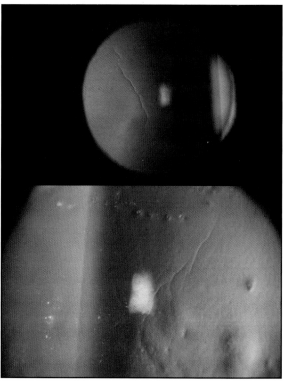

the first postoperative day. Close attention in this critical period pays off for the physician and patient, as the best outcomes are seen when significant striae are addressed within the first hours after surgery.

Several classification schemes have been used in the literature to describe the types of striae seen and to determine when intervention is needed. We find it is easiest to divide striae into two groups: those causing decreased visual acuity and those that are not visually significant. Striae that cause a decrease in visual acuity require treatment.

If noticed immediately after surgery (before the patient is discharged), we like to attempt to first smooth the flap at the slit-lamp using a lint-free sponge or cotton swab.[4] If this is unsuccessful, we take the patient back to the laser suite to refloat and realign the flap.

For striae that have been in place for longer periods, there are many ways to improve their effects:

- Refloating
- Hydration with hypotonic solution
- Stroking or smoothing
- Massaging
- Sandwich compression
- Flap suturing
- Epithelium removal
- Application of hyperthermic treatment
- Phototherapeutic keratectomy
- Discarding the flap with or without replacement lamellar keratoplasty

We have found that striae present longer than a few hours do not resolve completely with just refloating and realigning the flap (even those seen on postoperative day 1). For these chronic striae, our preferred method of treatment is as follows:

1. Scrape the epithelium from the central 80% of the flap (leaving the flap edge epithelium intact).
2. Lift the flap.
3. Overhydrate the flap with balanced salt solution.
4. Replace and realign the flap.
5. Place a bandage contact lens.

We feel strongly that epithelium removal is the key to successful treatment. Without this step, the striae in Bowman's layer and the underlying stroma remain locked in position by overlying epithelium.

Careful attention to technique and parameters at the time of LASIK can help prevent flap striae, but if you encounter this problem, you have options to treat and satisfy your patient.

References

1. Gimbel HV, Penno EE, van Westenbrugge JA, Ferensowicz M, Furlong MT. Incidence and management of intraoperative and early postoperative complications in 1000 consecutive laser in situ keratomileusis cases. *Ophthalmology.* 1998;105:1839-1847.
2. Neff KD, Probst LE. LASIK complications. In: Krachmer JH, Mannis MJ, Holland EJ, eds. *Cornea.* Philadelphia: Mosby Elsevier; 2011:1867-1869.
3. Choi CJ, Melki SA. Maddox rod effect to confirm the visual significance of laser in situ keratomileusis flap striae. *J Cataract Refract Surg.* 2011;37:1748-1750.
4. Solomon R, Donnenfeld ED, Perry HD, Doshi S, Biser S. Slitlamp stretching of the corneal flap after laser in situ keratomileusis to reduce corneal striae. *J Cataract Refract Surg.* 2003;29:1292-1296.

18
QUESTION

HOW DO I MANAGE PATIENTS WITH DRY EYES AFTER LASIK SURGERY?

Eric D. Donnenfeld, MD and Matthew J. Schear, DO

All patients experience at least transient dry eye following LASIK[1], and this is arguably the most common problem facing refractive surgeons today.[2-4] Following LASIK, the cornea overlying the flap is significantly anesthetic for 3 to 6 months.[2-4] As a result, all patients will have decreased tear production but may not realize it because of reduced corneal sensation. In general, only those patients whose eyes were dry or who were marginally compensated before surgery will have symptoms. Fortunately, the great majority of these symptoms resolve over a 2- to 4-week period after surgery.

There are several ways to reduce the likelihood of dry eye following LASIK. One of the most important preventative steps is to screen patients carefully prior to refractive surgery. Many who seek refractive surgery are actually preselected dry eye patients who are contact lens intolerant. Because these patients are uncomfortable wearing contact lenses due to their preexisting dry eye syndrome, they often seek LASIK for visual rehabilitation. In our opinion, mention of contact lens intolerance in the patient history should strongly suggest the possibility of underlying dry eye.

The dry eye history is perhaps the most important part of the LASIK work-up. We ask all patients whether they experience any eye symptoms, including sandy-gritty irritation, dryness, burning, or foreign body sensation. Carefully inspect the lids of patients who report morning eye irritation for signs of meibomitis, and pay close attention to the status of the meibomian gland orifices. Stenosis and closure of the meibomian glands, large palpebral fissure width, and decreased tear production all increase tear film osmolarity and cause dry eye. We perform basic tear testing including tear film break-up time (TBUT), look for tear debris in the inferior cul-de-sac, and perform Schirmer testing with anesthesia. Most important, we do supra-vital staining of the conjunctiva with lissamine green or rose bengal and fluorescein staining of the cornea to look for the classic staining pattern of dry eye (Figures 18-1 and 18-2). We have recently found tear osmolarity

Henderson BA, Yoo SH. *Curbside Consultation in Refractive and Lens-Based Surgery: 49 Clinical Questions* (pp 65-68)
© 2015 SLACK Incorporated

Figure 18-1. Supra-vital staining of the cornea with lissamine green demonstrating classic staining pattern of dry eye.

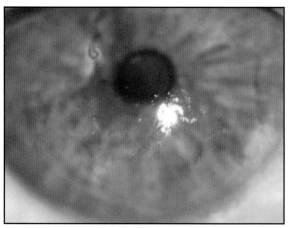

Figure 18-2. Rose bengal staining of the conjunctiva in a v-shaped distribution.

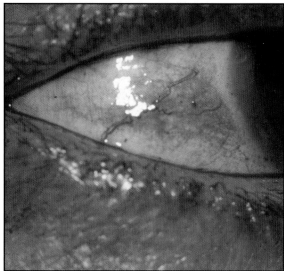

to be very helpful in identifying patients at risk for dry eye disease, and a new test that measures tear film MMP-9 levels shows great promise.

All patients with dry eye syndrome should be treated prior to LASIK surgery. Patients who have symptoms but no signs of corneal or conjunctival staining are generally excellent LASIK candidates. Patients with dry eye symptoms and mild conjunctival staining should be treated with therapeutic preservative-free artificial tears to stabilize the ocular surface prior to surgery. We consider corneal staining, on the other hand, to be a relative contraindication to surgery until the ocular surface has been stabilized. Patients with corneal staining are also treated with cyclosporine (CsA) 0.05%, therapeutic nonpreserved tears, lubricating ointment at night, and punctal occlusion. In patients who have meibomian gland disease (Figure 18-3), we add oral doxycycline 50 mg twice a day for 2 weeks and then daily for 1 additional month. We have also found that supplementation with the omega 3 fatty acids provided by eicosapentaenoic (EPA) and docosahexaenoic acid (DHA) is beneficial in cases of abnormal meibomian gland secretions and aqueous deficiency dry eye.

The role of inflammation in dry eye disease has been elucidated over the past decade. In patients seeking LASIK with moderate to severe dry eye, we pretreat with CsA 0.05% twice a day

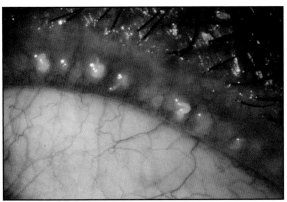

Figure 18-3. Meibomian gland inspissation.

for 3 months and then reassess dry eye status prior to considering surgery. Adding a low-dose corticosteroid such as loteprednol can improve dry eye signs and symptoms faster than cyclosporine alone. We recommend loteprednol 0.5% 4 times a day for 2 weeks prior to starting cyclosporine therapy, then taper down to twice a day for 2 weeks.

Intraoperative and Postoperative Management of LASIK

Preserving the corneal epithelium and preventing corneal abrasions intra- and postoperatively decreases the risk of dry eye. We minimize the use of topical anesthetics by giving the first dose when the patient enters the laser suite and the second dose immediately prior to surgery. The patients are instructed to close their eyes for 15 minutes before the flap is examined. In an attempt to promote epithelial healing and reduce the incidence of post-LASIK dry eye, we ask patients to keep their eyes closed for 4 hours after surgery and give them a structured schedule of artificial tear use. If the patient has symptoms of dry eye after LASIK, we insert inferior punctal plugs to stabilize the ocular surface; if the patient does not respond, we add oral doxycycline to the postoperative regimen. Many patients with meibomian gland disease also benefit from nutritional supplements containing omega-3 fatty acids. Finally, for patients who have long-term dry eye problems, we have found significant benefit from adding CsA 0.05% twice daily for 3 to 6 months.

Conclusion

One of the most common complications of LASIK surgery is dry eye. The incidence of post-LASIK dry eye can be reduced by identifying patients at risk for dry eye, maximizing tear film stability preoperatively, and minimizing risk of developing dry eye through intraoperative and postoperative therapeutic interventions. The risk of post-LASIK dry eye can be diminished with an intelligent surgical, pharmacologic, and behavioral approach to LASIK surgery. The surgeon should take appropriate steps at every stage of the surgical process to optimize the refractive outcome and minimize postoperative dry eye.

References

1. Toda I, Asano-Kato N, Hori-Komai Y, Tsubota K. Dry eye after laser in situ keratomileusis. *Am J Ophthalmol.* 2001;132(1):1-7.
2. Kanellopoulos AJ, Pallikaris IG, Donnenfeld ED, et al. Comparison of corneal sensation following photorefractive keratectomy and laser in situ keratomileusis. *J Cataract Refract Surg.* 1997;23(1):34-38.
3. Linna TU, Vesaluoma MH, Perez-Santonja JJ, et al. Effect of myopic LASIK on corneal sensitivity and morphology of subbasal nerves. *Invest Ophthalmol Vis Sci.* 2000;41(2):393-397.
4. Chuck RS, Quiros PA, Perez AC, McDonnell PJ. Corneal sensation after laser in situ keratomileusis. *J Cataract Refract Surg.* 2000;26(3):337-339.

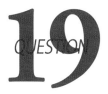

19

HOW DO I MANAGE PATIENTS WITH SEVERE GLARE SYMPTOMS AFTER LASIK?

Roberto Zaldivar, MD and Roger Zaldivar, MD

Glare can be defined as difficulty seeing in the presence of bright light. It was not uncommon to experience glare and halos in the early days of LASIK surgery. Moreover, night vision complaints such as starbusts, ghosting, and undefined optical phenomena were reported at rates of 10% to 60% in those days. Treatments were attempted at 3.5 to 4 mm with no transition zone with the untreated periphery of the cornea leading to a significant decrease in optical quality in mesopic vision caused by an increase of higher-order aberrations. The importance of treatment zones and setting lower refractive limits was not fully recognized.

Nowadays, with the advent of advanced LASIK treatments such as wavefront and aspheric profiles, treatment zones are being maximized and the attempt to over-ablate the peripheral cornea in order to blend the principal curvature of the optical zone smoothly into the peripheral cornea has markedly improved LASIK results and reduced the amount of visual complaints.

Despite the above-mentioned improvements in new generation lasers, peer-reviewed literature suggests that LASIK induces higher-order aberrations affecting contrast sensitivity as a result of changes in the corneal shape and cornea irregularities after the treatment.[1] The tear film plays a crucial role in achieving optimal quality of vision because it is the eye's first refractive surface. Its temporal disruption after LASIK induces dynamic microaberrations[2] that may be perceived as glare in certain situations. This tear reduction causes a temporal decrease in contrast sensitivity by scattering light in corneal irregularities. Other causes of persistent glare after LASIK surgery are residual refractive error, small optical zone related to pupil size, and a poorly centered ablation.[3]

Central corneal flattening after myopic correction affects the cornea's natural asphericity, turning the prolate corneal surface to oblate. The opposite happens in hyperopic profiles. These changes in corneal shape cause spherical aberration and astigmatism and are directly related to the pupil size because they tend to worsen in mesopic conditions due to pupil dilation.[3] This is

Henderson BA, Yoo SH. *Curbside Consultation in Refractive and Lens-Based Surgery: 49 Clinical Questions* (pp 69-72) © 2015 SLACK Incorporated

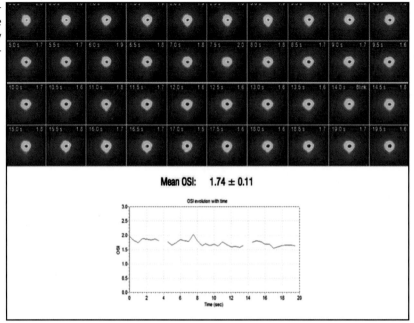

Figure 19-1. One-day postoperative tear film stability after phakic IOL surgery.

Mean OSI: 1.74 ± 0.11

described as a more intense perception of glare and halos around headlights and streetlights. In our practice, preoperative assessment of pupil size under different lighting conditions and not exceeding 6 diopters (D) of correction remains the standard of care. Special care must be taken in patients with more than 6 mm mesopic pupil and high attempted corrections (more than 7 D).

Clinical Assessment of Symptomatic Patients

The first and most important diagnostic step is to identify the location of the problem. This is an easy task in patients with aggressive myopic or hyperopic profiles with large mesopic pupils, but it can be a real threat in other cases. Regarding the analysis of tear film, the lack of correlation between signs and symptoms related to dry eye[4] and other optical phenomena such as spherical aberration makes our diagnosis unclear. We base our decision on two diagnostic techniques: ray-tracing aberrometry (iTrace) and double-pass technique (HD Analyzer; Visiometrics). We use aberrometry to evaluate the profile, centration, and induction of aberrations with different pupil conditions. The HD Analyzer gives us a complete sense of how the patient is imaging objects at the retina (Figure 19-1). It is the only device available that objectively measures the entire optical quality of the eye. It considers important information such as scattering and diffraction, which are underestimated by aberrometers based in Hartmann Shack and ray-tracing. The tear film quality and stability can be analyzed with the tear film analysis system.

Our first approach in patients with persistent glare symptoms after LASIK due to dry eye is administering fluorometholone 4 times daily plus artificial tears and gel at night for 1 month. If this does not improve the symptoms and we see a poor lacrimal meniscus, we suggest temporal intracanalicular punctum plugs to increase tear quantity and help surface restoration. If we determine that the patient's dissatisfaction is due to aberrations, lack of centration (Figure 19-2), or is related to a small optical zone in relation to the pupil size (Figure 19-3), we use brimonidine (Alphagan) or other soft pupil constrictor to decrease mesopic pupil size and diminish the symptomatology.

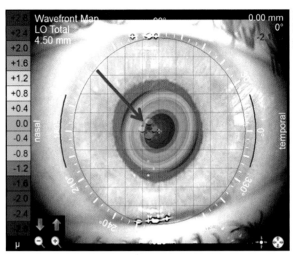

Figure 19-2. Assessment of centration with iTrace aberrometer. The red cross estimates the position of the line of sight.

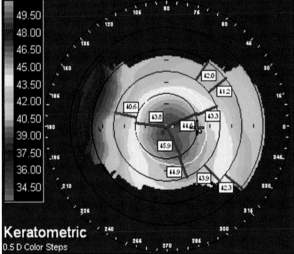

Figure 19-3. Small optical zone in hyperopic profile.

If the patient's symptoms improve after wearing spectacles, we infer that glare is originated because of residual error, so we do a retreatment as soon as we see a refractive stability.

Introducing an aspheric intraocular lens might be an option in patients with a previous aggressive myopic profile. It is important to point out that the crystalline lens tends to move from a negative spherical aberration when we are young to a positive spherical aberration as we age.

Neuroadaptation can help to make symptomatology less annoying through the next few months following the surgery, so it is always important to support the patient during the process. Time will help.

The Near Future

- With the advent of rotational dynamic eyetrackers, the chances of increasing eye aberrations are diminished. This revolutionary technology tracks the eye in x, y, and z directions, compensating for every micro-movement and allowing a more precise correction of higher-order aberrations.

- There will be better assessment of patients with potentially severe dry eye.
- Accurate osmolarity tests, Ocular Surface Disease Index score, biomicroscopy, Tear Film Analysis System, and appropriate chair time will help decrease dry eye complications after LASIK.
- Better and safer phakic intraocular lenses will decrease complications related to overablations.

References

1. Wang Y, Zhao KX, He JC, Jin Y, Zuo T. Ocular higher-order aberrations features analysis after corneal refractive surgery. *Chin Med J* (Engl). 2007;20;120(4):269-273.
2. Koh S, Maeda N, Hirohara Y, et al. Serial measurements of higher-order aberrations after blinking in normal subjects. *Invest Ophthalmol Vis Sci.* 2006;47(8):3318-3324.
3. Zhang J, Zhou YH, Li R, Tian L. Visual performance after conventional LASIK and wavefront-guided LASIK with iris-registration: Results at 1 year. *Int J Ophthalmol.* 2013;6(4):498-504.
4. Chan A, Manche EE. Effect of preoperative pupil size on quality of vision after wavefront-guided LASIK. *Ophthalmology.* 2011;118(4):736-741.
5. Nichols KK, Nichols JJ, Mitchell GL. The lack of association between signs and symptoms in patients with dry eye disease. *Cornea.* 2004;23(8):762-770.

HOW DO I MANAGE EPITHELIAL INGROWTH AFTER LASIK? WHAT IF IT RECURS?

Jorge L. Alió, MD, PhD and Alessandro Abbouda, MD

The reported incidence of epithelial ingrowth after LASIK varies from 0.2% to 12%, and increases to 32% after enhancements.[1] Epithelialization of the interface may occur as a result of two physiopathogenic mechanisms. In the first, corneal epithelium invades the interface at the periphery of the flap, most often after a bad coadaptation of the beveled edge of the inlay. In this case, circular whitish opacities are observed mainly at the periphery of the flap. The other mechanism involves epithelial cells planting beneath the flap and spreading during the course of the surgery. In these cases, the epithelial cells also appear as circular whitish opacities, but tend to concentrate closer to the visual axis. The epithelial ingrowth is asymptomatic during its initial phases, though very rarely, patients may complain of photophobia, foreign body sensation, or red eye. In advanced stages, patients complain of diminished visual acuity related to irregular astigmatism or visual symptoms such as glare, halos, or night visual disturbances attributable to a large growth at the periphery or growth of epithelial cells toward the center of the pupil. Careful slit-lamp examination of the flap borders, especially inferiorly with a superior hinge or temporally with a nasal hinge, may identify a fistula extending from the edge of the flap. Epithelial ingrowth may appear in two forms: small white or grayish spots or lines at the periphery (Figure 20-1) within 2 mm of the peripheral edge of the flap, or pearly islands of different sizes (Figure 20-2). If left untreated, the affected area of the flap disappears, the keratolysis progresses, and the growth spreads over the entire flap (Figure 20-3). Surgical treatment of epithelial ingrowth is very difficult and has a high incidence of recurrence.[1] Surgical treatment must be considered if (1) epithelial ingrowth progresses toward the visual axis and threatens best-corrected visual acuity; (2) epithelial ingrowth does not progress, but the cyst forms an elevation that causes irregular and uncorrectable astigmatism; or (3) the flap starts to melt. If there is a small nest of epithelium with a fistula at the edge, the best strategy is Nd:YAG treatment.[2] This can eliminate

Henderson BA, Yoo SH. *Curbside Consultation in Refractive*
and Lens-Based Surgery: 49 Clinical Questions (pp 73-76)
© 2015 SLACK Incorporated

Figure 20-1. (A) Small white spots (red arrow) and (B) grayish line of epithelial ingrowth (blue arrow).

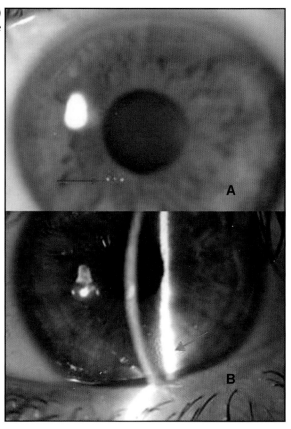

Figure 20-2. Pearl-like islands of different sizes of epithelial ingrowth (blue arrow) (aggressive form).

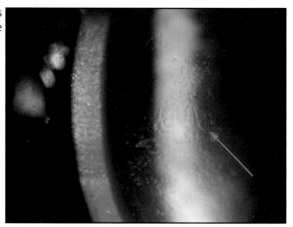

the source of the epithelium without lifting the flap. This technique uses a small spot size (8 μm) and minimal energy (0.6 mJ) first on the fistula area and then directly on the rest. An average of 10 to 40 pulses are emitted, depending on the size of the area to be treated. If the epithelial ingrowths reappear or the complication is very severe, other methods have been proposed.[3] In general, before the epithelium is broken, the border should be determined by microscopic inspection. If the border is not easily seen, apply gentle pressure to the limbus. If you have to lift the flap, break the epithelium at the junction, enter the interface with a thin spatula under the flap,

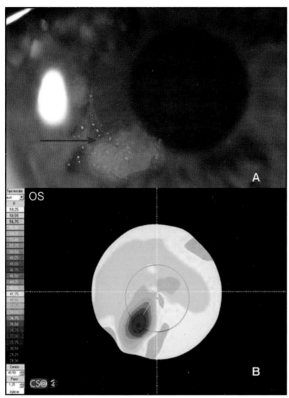

Figure 20-3. (A) Clinical aspect of melting stroma after epithelial ingrowth (red arrow) and (B) topographical appearance.

and then lift. Once the flap is up, the epithelial sheets must be removed by forceps if they detach easily, or by gentle scraping with a spatula and/or sponges. *Care must be taken not to reseed epithelial cells.* Of particular importance is to clean not only the stromal bed but also the stroma of the flap. Depending on the etiology of the disease, suturing the flap or a bandage contact lens may be important until the epithelium closes the wound and no cells are observed reappearing under the flap. An additional therapy to destroy epithelial cells is ethanol applied with a Merocel® sponge (Beaver-Visitec International, Ltd), which is then they are removed by careful washing with balanced salt solution; this procedure has a high risk of scarring. Excimer laser in the form of phototherapeutic keratectomy (PTK) may also be applied to the undersurface of the flap and the stromal bed to clean the invisible cells that remain after a careful cleaning. PTK of 10 microns has been advocated as the standard because deeper ablations may have undesirable refractive effects. Cryotherapy on both surfaces is another proposed method. Mitomycin C has also been used as a chemical suppressor of epithelial cells but was ineffective. When the flap is too irregular and too thin for extensive melting, a drastic treatment[4] is amputation and PTK with 0.02% mitomycin C. Compensatory epithelial hyperplasia then smoothes the surface in the short term and, over 2 to 3 years, the cornea itself also can undergo remodeling. Finally, extensive research has been done on drops that could remove cells from the interface without the need to lift the flap.[3]

References

1. Gimbel HV, Penno EE, Van Westenbrugge JA, et al. Incidence and management of intraoperative and early post-operative complications in 1000 consecutive laser in situ keratomileusis cases. *Ophthalmology*. 1998;105:1839-1847.

2. Ayala M, Alió JL, Mulet ME, De La Hoz F. Treatment of laser in situ keratomileusis interface epithelial ingrowth with neodymium:yytrium–aluminum–garnet laser. *Am J Ophthalmol*. 2008;145:630-634.

3. Tamayo GE. Epithelial ingrowth. In: Alió JL, Azar D, eds. *Management of Complications in Refractive Surgery*. Berlin Heidelberg: Springer Verlag; 2008.

4. Duffey R. A drastic cure for poor follow up. *Eyenet*. 2012;48-49. Available at: http://www.aao.org/publications/eyenet/201209/upload/September-2012-Feature.pdf.

How Do I Manage Severe Haze After Photorefractive Keratectomy?

Florence Cabot, MD and Sonia H. Yoo, MD

Corneal haze is an overreaction of remaining keratocytes affecting epithelium and anterior stroma that may last for months to years after surgery (Figure 21-1). Severity depends on duration of the epithelial defect and depth of the stromal injury. Preoperative high ametropia, requiring a deep corneal ablation, is the major risk factor for developing haze after photorefractive keratectomy (PRK). Other risk factors include heavy ultraviolet light exposure, prior corneal surgery, and persistent epithelial defects. In particular, patients who have had corneal surgeries such as LASIK, corneal transplant, and radial keratotomy have increased risk of haze relative to virgin corneas.[1]

When treating severe haze, we would first recommend aggressive administration of topical corticosteroids and lubricating drops. We use prednisolone acetate 1% drops administered 8 times per day, tapering the steroids slowly over 3 to 4 months. If the haze decreases and best corrected visual acuity improves but more corticosteroid therapy is required, we switch to fluorometholone drops and taper over several weeks to several months to avoid steroid dependence and related complications (early cataract, increasing intraocular pressure, and especially pressure-induced steroid keratitis, which can lead to glaucoma).[2]

When haze does not respond to steroid treatment, there are two options, both using adjuvant 0.02% mitomycin C (MMC). The first approach consists of manually scraping the epithelium and the subepithelial anterior stromal haze.[3] It is very important to remove as much scar tissue as possible because the MMC will inhibit new scar formation only. A corneal sponge is soaked with 0.02% MMC and placed on the corneal surface for 2 minutes. The eye is then irrigated with copious balanced saline solution (BSS) and a bandage contact lens is placed to aid in patient comfort while the epithelium heals. The postoperative treatment includes antibiotic/steroid and nonsteroidal drops.

Henderson BA, Yoo SH. *Curbside Consultation in Refractive and Lens-Based Surgery: 49 Clinical Questions* (pp 77-78)
© 2015 SLACK Incorporated

Figure 21-1. Slit-lamp photo of a mild central corneal haze.

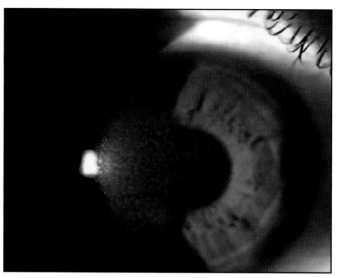

The second option involves phototherapeutic keratectomy (PTK).[4] In this procedure, most surgeons prefer a transepithelial PTK approach. This is performed in a dark room with the microscope light low enough to visualize the natural epithelial and haze fluorescence, allowing accurate visualization of the breakthrough point of the "epithelium and haze" (blue fluorescence) onto normal stroma (black). Some surgeons add simultaneous PRK to correct the usual refractive regression associated with haze. After the laser treatment, an 8-mm sponge soaked in 0.02% MMC is applied directly over the area of haze for 2 minutes. The surface of the cornea is then thoroughly irrigated with BSS. At the end of the procedure, a bandage soft contact lens is placed and antibiotic drops and prednisolone acetate 1% are applied 4 times per day for 1 week; thereafter, the antibiotic is discontinued and steroids tapered over 1 to 3 months. Some surgeons consider PTK to be more precise than manual scraping because it leaves a smoother surface, free of any microscopic islands of remaining scar tissue.

Ultimately, the best treatment for haze is prevention. Adjunctive use of prophylactic MMC has significantly reduced the incidence of post-PRK haze in high-risk cases. Surgeons should advise patients undergoing PRK to avoid excessive sun exposure, which is associated with the development of haze.[1] Fortunately, with the use of modern excimer lasers, clinically significant haze is now uncommon.

References

1. Trattler W, Barnes S. Current trends in advanced surface ablation. *Curr Opin Ophthalmol.* 2008;19:330-334.
2. Arshinoff SA, Mills MD, Haber S. Pharmacotherapy of photorefractive keratectomy. *J Cataract Refract Surg.* 1996;22(8):1037-1044.
3. Majmudar PA, Forstot L, Dennis RF, et al. Topical mitomycin-C for subepithelial fibrosis after refractive corneal surgery. *Ophthalmology.* 2000;107:89-94.
4. Lee YG, Chen WY, Petroll WM, et al. Corneal haze after photorefractive keratectomy using different epithelial removal techniques: Mechanical debridement versus laser scrape. *Ophthalmology.* 2001;108(1):112-120.

HOW DO I DETECT AND MANAGE ECTASIA AFTER LASIK?

Rosane de Oliveira Corrêa, MD; Renato Ambrósio Jr, MD, PhD; and William Trattler, MD

Post-LASIK ectasia is an uncommon but serious complication of laser vision correction.[1] Ectasia is characterized by progressive steepening of the cornea and irregular astigmatism that may cause severe impairment of the visual acuity, leading to the need for contact lenses, and in some cases, therapeutic procedures such as Intacs or keratoplasty.[1,2] Since it was first reported by Theo Seiler in 1996, improvements in refractive screenings and innovations in surgical techniques have been developed and corneal ectasia incidence has been declining. However, the condition still occurs and represents the major concern among experts.[1,2]

Ectasia after LASIK might occur in a few days to years after the procedure, most commonly in eyes with abnormal corneal shape such as forme fruste keratoconus (FFKC), keratoconus, or pellucid marginal degeneration. In addition, some patients with very mild corneal shape abnormalities can develop post-LASIK ectasia. Potential risk factors include age, thin corneas in association with abnormal corneal shape, thin residual stromal bed (due to thick flap or higher corrections), eye rubbing, and family history of keratoconus.[1,3-6] One of the landmark papers on this topic was written by Randleman et al and published in 2003, where for the first time a series of post-LASIK ectasia cases were compared with a control group.[7] The study revealed that FFKC was a major risk factor for post-LASIK ectasia because 88% of the eyes with ectasia had preoperative FFKC, while only 3% of the 200 control eyes who had LASIK at Emory were identified as having FFKC preoperatively. Interestingly, cases with no identified risk factors preoperatively have been described.[3-6] The lamellar cut effect combined with excimer laser ablation generates a biomechanical impact that can culminate in chronic biomechanical failure of the insufficient residual stromal bed (RSB). Subsequently, progressive thinning and bulging of the cornea leads to a myopic shift and irregular astigmatism, resulting in reduced uncorrected and best-corrected visual acuity (UCVA and BCVA).[1,3]

Henderson BA, Yoo SH. *Curbside Consultation in Refractive and Lens-Based Surgery: 49 Clinical Questions* (pp 79-83)
© 2015 SLACK Incorporated

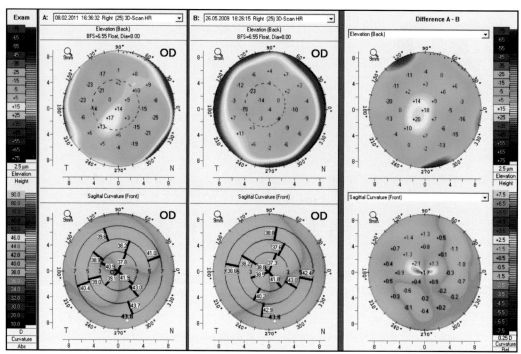

Figure 22-1. Difference maps from posterior elevation (top) and anterior curvature (bottom) of a patient who had LASIK in 2004 for OD. There is a significant early change on the posterior elevation difference map: +20 µm (top). Note that the progressive early change in posterior elevation is more evident than in anterior curvature (bottom). For follow-up comparison, best-fit sphere should have the same reference shape in all exams (BFS fixed 8-mm zone diameter and 6.55 mm of radius of curvature).

Our routine in identifying patients with early ectasia after LASIK includes complete eye exam (UCVA, BCVA, manifest refraction, slit-lamp examination, ocular surface evaluation, intraocular pressure, and retina exam), corneal topography and tomography, biomechanical assessment, and total ocular aberrometry. Other conditions such as dry eye should be excluded.

Progressive displacement of the posterior corneal elevation demonstrated by corneal tomography or forward protrusion observed in Placido topography is an early sign of ectasia.[8] However, anterior curvature alone may not supply enough data to detect subclinical disease (Figure 22-1). We evaluated a 36-year-old woman who had LASIK in the right eye (OD) in 2004: preoperative manifest refraction spherical equivalent was –2.50 sphere and flap thickness measurement was 215 µm. Progressive decreasing in BCVA and astigmatic shift, from 20/25 (–0.25 sphere –1.25 cyl 54 degrees) to 20/40 (-0.25 sphere –3.00 cyl 60 degrees), was detected, along with a significant early change on the posterior elevation difference map (+20 µm) 7 years after LASIK (see Figure 22-1). Measuring corneal posterior elevation with Pentacam (Oculus) provides an accurate representation of the true shape of the cornea not influenced by insufficiency of the tear film or the use of lubricant drops.[3,8] However, proper alignment of the corneal surfaces and correct measurements (scans with quality specification graded as "ok") are crucial to prevent artifacts from affecting the corneal maps evaluation.[1,8] For postoperative follow-up comparison, elevation maps should have identical reference body (same fixed corneal zone diameter and radius of curvature in all exams [see Figure 22-1]).[1,8] Given the fact that a normal cornea has a prolate surface and 8- to 9-mm zone ranges, a reference surface that allows for subtle ectatic disease identification, setting best-fit sphere (BFS) in an 8-mm zone diameter is recommended.[1,8] Larger zones yielding a flatter BFS and toric ellipsoid surface as a reference body could mask ectatic area detection.[1,8]

Prevention is the best strategy because ectasia is difficult to manage.[5-9] Detecting patients who may be at risk preoperatively using appropriate screening and operating on good candidates with proper surgical technique plays a very important role.[1,3,5-8] Sub-Bowman's keratomileusis with femtosecond laser has been demonstrated to be a safer technique, avoiding corneal ectasia and other complications when compared with traditional femtosecond flaps and flaps created by mechanical microkeratome.[8] Uniform, thin, planar flaps created by femtosecond laser have better predictability of the flap thickness and appear to lead to greater biomechanical stability.[8] Applying intraoperative ultrasonic pachymetry just after the flap is lifted is a helpful tool and can also predict risk for ectasia by helping identify eyes with a deeper than expected flap.[8]

Understanding how the ectatic process happened is critical for management. When evaluating a patient with post-LASIK ectasia, it is important to investigate clinical data and tomographic and biomechanic corneal susceptibility on LASIK preoperative evaluation. Risk factors related to surgical technique may be studied by assessing flap and RSB thickness with a Scheimpflug image or high-resolution optical coherence tomography (OCT). Ocular surface optimization is necessary and includes preservative-free lubricant drops, nutritional supplementation with omega 3 essential fatty acids, topical cyclosporine, and punctal plug. Avoiding eye rubbing and lowering ocular pressure may decrease the risk for progression of the disease.[2]

Spectacles or contact lenses are first-line treatment and might improve visual acuity in early ectatic corneas.[2] As the ectatic process advances, using wavefront measurements can help with determining the optimal spectacle correction.[9]

As the disease progresses to advanced irregular astigmatism, corrective lenses no longer provide satisfactory vision.[2] Intrastromal corneal ring segment (ICRS) implants have been indicated for patients with contact lens intolerance and RSB thickness more than 300 microns, postponing corneal transplant. ICRS is safe and potentially reversible and works well when using the femtosecond laser to create the channels.[10,11] ICRS presents a mechanical effect and acts as additional tissue into the corneal stroma, resulting in corneal flattening. Previous studies report improvement in visual acuity, keratometric parameters, and biomechanical characteristics following ICRS.

Corneal crosslinking (CXL) is a unique treatment to stop progression of corneal ectatic disorders, making the cornea stronger and stiffer.[12] Application of riboflavin drops with the epithelium left intact (Epi-ON) followed by ultraviolet UVA light has been our practice and has proved to be an effective and safe technique with less pain, rapid healing, and a very low risk for adverse effects when compared to epithelium-off CXL techniques.[12] In our study (CXL-USA), transepithelial CXL was able to halt progressive vision loss and improve at least 1 line of UCVA and BCVA in 50% of eyes at 1 year follow-up.[13] Corneal CXL can be performed along with phakic intraocular lens implant or customized photorefractive keratectomy (PRK) to reduce refractive errors.[14] We reported a 29-year-old female patient with post-LASIK ectasia and flap thickness of 199 µm on corneal OCT (Figure 22-2A) in the left eye (OS), who had undergone topography-guided PRK combined with collagen CXL in the same day (Athens Protocol).[14] The patient has demonstrated improvement in BCVA from 20/40 (+2.50 sphere –3.25 cyl 94 degrees) to 20/25 (+1.0 sphere), by reducing irregular astigmatism and stabilizing the ectatic process as evidenced on tomographic maps (Figure 22-2B and 22-2C).

Identifying corneas at risk preoperatively is the most effective strategy in preventing post-LASIK ectasia. Refractive screenings, including Placido topography, corneal tomography, biomechanical analysis, and epithelial map using corneal OCT, are potential technologies to help identify corneas at risk for ectasia and to help select good candidates properly.

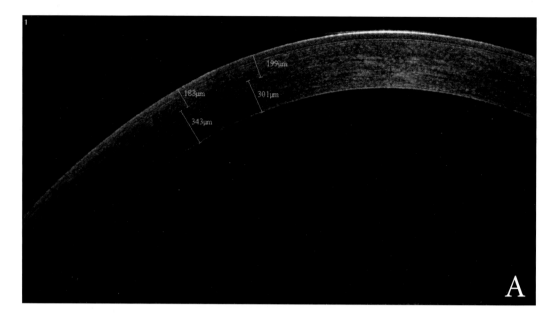

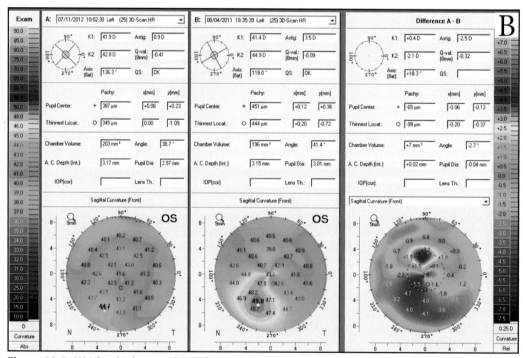

Figure 22-2. (A) Ultra-high corneal OCT from OS showing an irregular flap thickness of 199 μm and RSB thickness of 301 μm in the paracentral cornea. Flap seems to be thicker in the central cornea. (B) Post-LASIK ectasia management in the OS. After performing PRK combined with corneal CXL in the same day (Athens Protocol), there was a significant improvement in BSCVA and in astigmatism, which could be evidenced by anterior curvature difference A-B map (A-B, post- and pre-treatment, respectively). *(continued)*

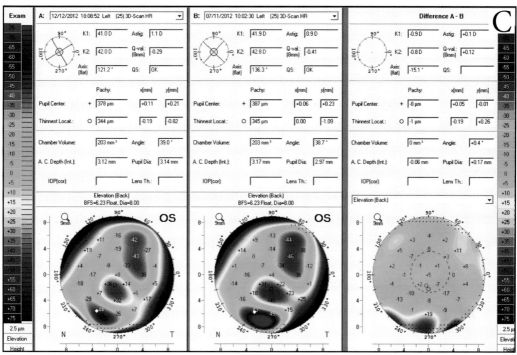

Figure 22-2 (continued). (C) The same case report showing ectasia stability on the posterior elevation map. BFS should have the same fixed shape in sequential exams.

References

1. Binder PS, Lindstrom RL, Stulting RD, et al. Keratoconus and corneal ectasia after LASIK. *J Refract Surg.* 2005;2:749-752.
2. Ambrósio R Jr, Jardim D, Neto MV, Wilson S. Management of unsuccessful LASIK surgery. *Compr Ophthalmol Update.* 2007;8(3):125-131.
3. Wang JC, Hufnagel TJ, Buxton DF. Bilateral keractesia after unilateral laser in situ keratomileusis: A retrospective diagnosis of ectatic corneal disorder. *J Cataract Refract Surg.* 2003;29(10):2015-2018.
4. Randleman JB. Evaluating risk factors for ectasia: What is the goal of assessing risk? *J Refract Surg.* 2010;26:236-237.
5. Binder PS, Trattler WB. Evaluation of a risk factor scoring system for corneal ectasia after LASIK in eyes with normal topography. *J Refract Surg.* 2010;26:241-250.
6. Ambrósio R Jr, Dawson DG, Salomao M, Guerra FP, Caiado AL, Belin MW. Corneal ectasia after LASIK despite low preoperative risk: Tomographic and biomechanical findings in the unoperated, stable, fellow eye. *J Refract Surg.* 2010;26:906-911.
7. Randleman JB, Russell B, Ward MA, et al. Risk factors and prognosis for corneal ectasia after LASIK. *Ophthalmology.* 2003;110:267-275.
8. Grewal DS, Brar GS, Grewal SPS. Posterior corneal elevation after LASIK with three flap techniques as measured by Pentacam. *J Refract Surg.* 2011;27(4):261-268.
9. Belin MW, Khachikian SS, Ambrósio R Jr, Salomao M. Keratoconus/ectasia detection with the Oculus Pentacam: Belin Ambrósio ectasia display. *Highlights of Ophthalmology.* 2007;35(6):5-12.
10. Ambrósio R Jr. Intrastromal Corneal Ring Segments for Keratoconus: Results and Correlation with Preoperative Corneal Biomechanics. 39o Varilux Award 2010-2011, Brazilian Ophthalmology Society Congress.
11. Ertan A, Colin J. Intracorneal rings for keratoconus and keractasia. *J Cataract Refract Surg.* 2007;33(7):1303-1314.
12. Rubinfeld R. CXL with the epithelium on or off: Which is better? *Cataract & Refractive Surgery Today,* May 2012.
13. Rubinfeld R, Trattler W, Forstot L, et al. Retrospective evaluation of epithelial–on cross-linking (CXL). Poster accepted for the American Academy of Ophthalmology Annual Meeting, November 11, 2012, Chicago, IL.
14. Kanellopoulos AJ, Binder PS. Management of corneal ectasia after LASIK with combined, same-day, topography-guided partial transepithelial PRK and collagen cross-linking: The Athens protocol. *J Refract Surg.* 2011;27(5):323-331.

23

QUESTION

AFTER AN INCOMPLETE FLAP AND ABORTED LASIK, HOW AND WHEN DO I MANAGE THE RESIDUAL REFRACTIVE ERROR? PRK WITH OR WITHOUT MMC, LASIK, OR CONTACT LENS?

Michael C. Knorz, MD

After cutting an incomplete flap, I wait for at least 3 months to let the cornea heal. If the complication occurred in the first eye, the patient can simply continue wearing glasses during this time. If the complication occurred in the second eye, the problem of anisometropia has to be addressed. Up to 2 diopters (D) poses no problem, but for higher corrections, I advise the patient to use a soft contact lens to correct his or her refractive error starting no sooner than 2 weeks after surgery.

I prefer to perform LASIK again as long as the initial flap was not thicker than about 120 µm. If possible, I measure the thickness of the first flap with optical coherence tomography (OCT). I use a femtosecond laser and program a flap thickness 50 µm thicker than the first flap. This is because the gas bubbles created by the femtosecond laser may otherwise re-open the incomplete first cut. The minimum difference between the two cuts is 50 µm if a femtosecond laser is used. If a mechanical microkeratome is used, the second cut should also be deeper than the first one, but the difference does not have to be 50 µm, just use a thicker flap than the initial one. Published results of re-cuts with mechanical microkeratomes are good.[1]

I perform surface ablation if the first flap's thickness cannot be measured, the first flap was thicker than 120 µm, or the surgery was performed elsewhere and clear data are unavailable. I use alcohol to remove the epithelium because mechanical removal may interfere with the incomplete flap. Do not use a brush, as this can dislodge the first flap! I also prefer surface ablation if there is visible scarring in the cornea because this might interfere with the femtosecond laser or if the cornea is thinner than 500 µm. If available, transepithelial photorefractive keratectomy (PRK) is also an excellent option to retreat incomplete flaps. In any case, when using surface ablation, I will also use mitomycin C (0.2% for 20 sec), as I do routinely in any retreatment done on the surface (eg, PRK after LASIK, or PRK after PRK).[2]

Henderson BA, Yoo SH. *Curbside Consultation in Refractive and Lens-Based Surgery: 49 Clinical Questions* (pp 85-86)
© 2015 SLACK Incorporated

Although I prefer LASIK, I believe surface ablation is the safer option if there is any doubt about the previous surgery (flap thickness, regularity). The disadvantages are reduced patient comfort and longer visual recovery.

References

1. Ito M, Hori-Komai Y, Tsubota K. Risk factors and retreatment results of intraoperative flap complications in LASIK. *J Cataract Refract Surg.* 2004;30:1240-1247.
2. Santiago MR, Netto MV, Wilson SE. Mitomicin C: Biological effects and its use in refractive surgery. *Cornea.* 2012;31:311-321.

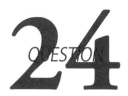

A PATIENT HAD LASIK 10 YEARS AGO AND WANTS RETREATMENT FOR RESIDUAL REFRACTIVE ERROR. HOW SHOULD I PROCEED?

Sumitra S. Khandelwal, MD and Elizabeth A. Davis, MD, FACS

Refractive enhancements are performed in 3% to 10% of eyes following primary myopic LASIK and 20% to 30% after primary hyperopic LASIK. When considering an enhancement, proper examination and appropriate patient counseling are essential.

History

A good history includes preoperative data from the primary LASIK, including corneal topography, subjective outcomes following the surgery, and the current complaints of the patient. For example, a patient in his or her 40s who notices blurry vision when reading may be an emerging presbyope. A patient complaining of glare or difficulty with night driving may have higher-order aberrations, an early cataract, or a residual refractive error. A patient who has fluctuating vision may have poor tear film stability due to dry eye or meibomian gland dysfunction. Meanwhile, a patient who describes vision that was never as good in one eye as the other after LASIK may have had under- or overcorrection; flap issues such as striae, epithelial ingrowth (Figure 24-1), or buttonhole; or other pathology such as irregular astigmatism, decentration, or ectasia. Ask specifically for any history suggestive of amblyopia in case of asymmetric visual recovery.

Clinical Exam

A careful clinical exam starts with uncorrected visual acuity (UCVA) and best-corrected distance visual acuity (BCVA) with manifest refraction. A complete eye exam includes, but is not

Henderson BA, Yoo SH. *Curbside Consultation in Refractive and Lens-Based Surgery: 49 Clinical Questions* (pp 87-91)
© 2015 SLACK Incorporated

Figure 24-1. Significant epithelial ingrowth following flap lift. The primary surgery was 5 years prior. The patient developed irregular astigmatism and paracentral ingrowth requiring flap lift, debridement, and fibrin glue.

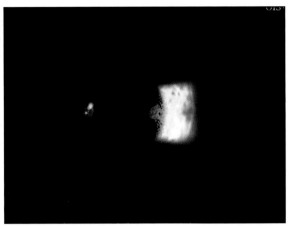

limited to, eye dominance, extraocular movements, intraocular pressure, manual keratometry, topography, and pachymetry, all of which should be documented. Slit-lamp examination includes any signs of dry eye and blepharitis. Examination of the cornea should look for anterior basement dystrophy or flap irregularities. Any lens findings should be noted, even if early in nature. A thorough posterior segment examination should be documented. Perform corneal topography to look for centration of ablation, thinnest pachymetry, and any irregular astigmatism. Optical coherence tomography (OCT) should be performed to quantify the primary LASIK flap thickness.

Treatment

The options for enhancement after LASIK include flap lift, flap recut, and surface ablation. The risk of epithelial ingrowth is higher in flaps lifted more than 3 years after primary surgery.[1] With flap recutting, the planes of the old and new flaps can intersect, leaving misplaced tissue fragments that can induce irregular astigmatism.

We prefer surface ablation on all enhancements. Epithelial removal is performed with 70% ethanol. After the ablation, 0.02% mitomycin C (MMC) is applied for 12 seconds in most cases. Some surgeons advocate reducing ablations by 10% when using MMC.

Patients should be counseled about the expectations of discomfort, contact lens placement, and speed of visual recovery after photorefractive keratectomy (PRK), as opposed to primary LASIK. Patients undergoing PRK after LASIK may experience some stromal haze even with MMC; this improves with topical steroids and is rarely visually significant. If a patient had stromal haze following primary PRK, we will often increase the duration of the MMC application.

There are a few special situations to consider in evaluating for enhancement:

- Hyperopic regression: Regression is more common in hyperopic patients. In addition, mild hyperopic outcomes after primary LASIK may not become apparent until patients become presbyopic. Early hyperopic regression is likely due to peripheral epithelial hyperplasia in response to central corneal steeping. It is important not to chase the hyperopic shift and create more central steepening. In general, we consider treatments to be additive; we prefer the total cumulative amount of hyperopic ablation performed to be less than 4 diopters (D) (Figure 24-2).

- Ectasia: Patients who have increasing myopia and/or astigmatism following LASIK may be experiencing LASIK ectasia. Clinical signs include keratometric steepening, corneal thinning, and loss of UCVA and BCVA. Corneal topography is usually diagnostic. Preoperative risk

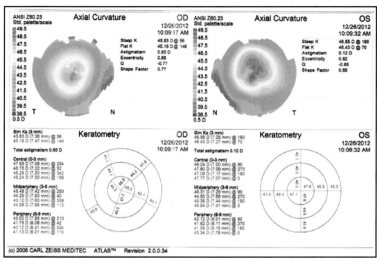

Figure 24-2. Example of hyperopic LASIK. The patient's preoperative data were not known, so a decision was made to postpone surgery until his amount of primary hyperopic treatment was determined using his previous surgical records.

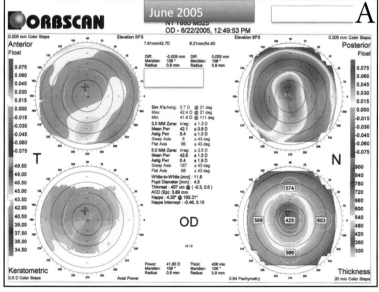

Figure 24-3. (A) Sequence of topography of a patient with ectasia after LASIK. Postoperative topography 8 years after myopic LASIK. The patient presented with symptoms of ghosting and decreased vision with a BCVA of 20/20 and a refraction of $-1.75 + 0.75 \times 020$. Topography shows inferior steepening and enhancement was deferred. *(continued)*

factors include abnormal topography, low residual stromal bed, younger age, and a thinner preoperative cornea.

- ○ The surgeon should be wary of new, induced astigmatism or loss of BCVA. Regression is rarely as high as the primary refractive error and such a finding is concerning. Data from before the primary surgery are useful but difficult to obtain at times (Figure 24-3). In these cases, topography is essential in determining whether the patient is a good candidate for an enhancement.

- Presbyopia: If a patient in the presbyopic age range is able to read without glasses and requests enhancement in a myopic eye, it is important to discuss the immediate loss of near vision that will occur. If both eyes have a mild myopic shift, we offer monovision for these patients by correcting the dominant eye to plano and leaving the nondominant eye myopic.

Figure 24-3 (continued).
(B) Topography 2 years later with BCVA 20/25 with worsening cylinder. (C) Topography 2 years later with worsening crab claw appearance and a BCVA of 20/40.

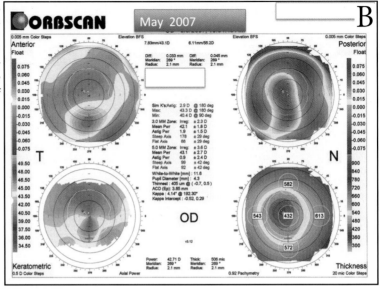

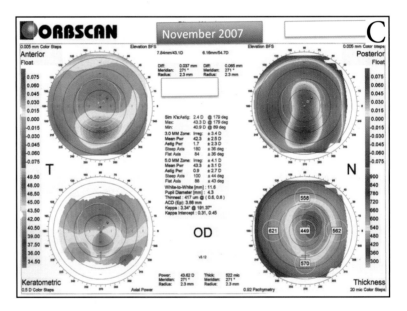

- Early cataracts: A myopic shift may be due to nuclear sclerosis, and a careful lens examination should be performed. In a patient who has a cataract that is not yet visually significant, a discussion of natural lens extraction rather than corneal refractive surgery may be appropriate.

Conclusion

A patient who requests an enhancement after primary LASIK should be evaluated carefully to determine whether he or she is a good candidate and counseled appropriately.

References

1. Caster AI, Friess DW, Schwendeman FJ. Incidence of epithelial ingrowth in primary and retreatment laser in situ keratomileusis. *J Cataract Refract Surg.* 2010;36(1):97-101.
2. Davis EA, Hardten DR, Lindstrom M, Samuelson TW, Lindstrom RL. LASIK enhancements: A comparison of lifting to recutting the flap. *Ophthalmology.* 2002;109(12):2308-2313.
3. Güell JL, Elies D, Gris O, Manero F, Morral M. Femtosecond laser-assisted enhancements after laser in situ keratomileusis. *J Cataract Refract Surg.* 2011;37(11):1928-1931.
4. Randleman JB, Woodward M, Lynn MJ, Stulting RD. Risk assessment for ectasia after corneal refractive surgery. *Ophthalmology.* 2008;115(1):37-50.

SECTION IV

REFRACTIVE
CATARACT SURGERY

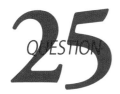

QUESTION 25

IF A PATIENT HAS HAD PREVIOUS CORNEAL REFRACTIVE SURGERY, WHAT TYPE OF IOL WOULD YOU CHOOSE? DOES IT MATTER IF IT WAS MYOPIC OR HYPEROPIC CORNEAL REFRACTIVE SURGERY?

Edward C. Lai, MD and Jessica B. Ciralsky, MD

Corneal refractive surgery in the United States dates back to 1978 with the introduction of radial keratotomy (RK). In the mid-1990s, photorefractive keratectomy (PRK) received Food and Drug Administration (FDA) approval, followed by LASIK only a few years later. Now that over 30 years have passed since the first refractive procedures were performed, many of these patients are developing cataracts and undergoing cataract surgery. This population of patients pursued refractive surgery with high expectations, and for the majority of these patients, those expectations were met. Similar outcomes are now being expected from cataract surgery, including the desire for spectacle and contact lens independence, the same motivation that drove the refractive surgery market.

Corneal refractive surgery, however, has physically changed the cornea, making intraocular lens (IOL) calculations and selection more difficult. Improved methods and formulas have been developed and refined over the last few years to increase the predictability of IOL calculations. Nevertheless, residual refractive errors are still common in this population and refractive surgery enhancements are often necessary to achieve emmetropia.

Higher-order aberrations, particularly spherical aberration, are also altered by corneal refractive surgery. Traditional non-wavefront PRK or LASIK induces higher-order aberrations. Eyes with increased levels of higher-order aberrations have reduced contrast sensitivity and decreased visual quality, particularly in mesopic conditions. Newer excimer lasers have been designed using wavefront-guided or wavefront-optimized technology to minimize the induction of higher-order aberrations; however, these aberrations have not been completely eliminated.

The spherical aberration of the cornea is inherently positive, averaging +0.27 µm. Myopic PRK or LASIK typically produces positive spherical aberrations, compounding the already positive

Henderson BA, Yoo SH. *Curbside Consultation in Refractive and Lens-Based Surgery: 49 Clinical Questions* (pp 95-97)
© 2015 SLACK Incorporated

corneal sphericity. Hyperopic PRK or LASIK, on the other hand, generally creates negative spherical aberrations, counteracting the positive corneal sphericity. These induced aberrations tend to increase with larger amounts of correction. The natural crystalline lens also contributes to the overall sphericity of the eye. With cataract surgery and the introduction of an IOL, the overall sphericity of the eye can be modified. Traditional IOLs are spherical, further contributing to the positive sphericity of the eye. Most new IOLs are also available on an aspheric platform and induce either zero or negative amounts of sphericity. An ideal IOL should aim to neuralize the corneal and minimize the eye's total sphericity.

An individual eye's sphericity can be measured with an aberrometer, and IOLs can be specifically chosen to offset the exact amount of sphericity in an individual eye. However, after refractive surgery, the cornea's sphericity can vary widely and it is often difficult to find a lens with the exact spherical aberration required for the best image quality. It is also important to note that actual sphericity of an IOL depends on its power. Alternatively, IOLs can be chosen based on a patient's ocular history. If a patient previously had myopic refractive surgery, we choose an aspheric lens to counteract the positive sphericity that is both inherent in the cornea and induced by the treatment. In general, we feel most patients with previous myopic refractive surgery benefit from IOLs with higher amounts of negative asphericity. For patients with previous hyperopic refractive surgery, we would choose either a zero sphericity lens or a spherical lens to balance the negative sphericity induced by the treatment.

Toric lenses can be considered for patients with residual corneal astigmatism. It is important to check topography to ensure the astigmatism is symmetrical and regular. Ruling out irregular astigmatism or postrefractive ectasia is essential. We have rarely had to implant a toric lens in a post-PRK or LASIK patient because we typically find that most of the astigmatism is well treated by the initial refractive surgery. We generally avoid toric lens implantation in post-RK patients because the astigmatism is often unstable and progressive.

The utility of an accommodating lens in a postrefractive patient has been poorly studied to date, but the combination of a monofocal platform and presbyopia correction is attractive in this population of patients, especially in those with traditional non-wavefront ablations. We have successfully implanted accommodating lenses in many patients who are post-PRK or LASIK with good results. The only accommodating lens currently available in the United States comes in several different models. We choose the aspheric version for post-myopic treatments and the spherical platform for post-hyperopic treatments. We typically avoid implanting this lens in post-RK patients given the unpredictability of the lens calculation and the small 5-mm optical zone, which may induce more glare in these patients.

Implantation of multifocal lenses in postrefractive patients has been met with resistance due to the possibility of creating additional symptoms of glare, halos, and reduced contrast sensitivity. Many surgeons will altogether avoid implanting multifocal lenses in patients treated with non-wavefront ablations. Additionally, there is the difficulty of predicting the lens power in a population with a low tolerance for residual refractive error. However, the motivation in these patients to achieve spectacle independence is very high. Several published studies have compared visual quality after previous hyperopic or myopic LASIK with phakic controls.[1,2] Both studies showed slightly worse visual performance in mesopic conditions when a spherical multifocal was implanted; for the post-myopic LASIK patients, these results improved when an aspheric platform was chosen. Therefore, we choose aspheric platforms for post-myopic patients and spherical platforms for post-hyperopic treatments. We completely avoid multifocals in my post-RK patients. We tend to only implant multifocal lenses in highly motivated postrefractive patients who are able and willing to undergo a laser enhancement, if necessary, and fully understand the risks and potential benefits. We always plan ahead for the possibility of a postoperative laser enhancement.

Millions of patients have undergone refractive surgery over the past 3 decades. IOL selection in these postrefractive patients is challenging on many fronts. The inaccuracy of IOL calculations often leaves patients with residual refractive errors, making the selection of a presbyopic-correcting lens more problematic. Refractive enhancements are often necessary and must be planned for ahead of time. Additionally, the eye's overall higher-order aberrations can be worsened by the specific lens chosen. Fortunately, as IOL technology continues to evolve, patient results continue to improve. Hopefully, future studies will help establish guidelines for ideal IOL selection for each patient. As always, the importance of counseling patients on the goals of surgery and the ability to reach those goals is paramount.

References

1. Alfonso JF, Fernández-Vega L, Baamonde B, Madrid-Costa D, Montés-Micó R. Visual quality after diffractive intraocular lens implantation in eyes with previous hyperopic laser in situ keratomileusis. *J Cataract Refract Surg.* 2011;37(6):1090-1096.
2. Fernández-Vega L, Madrid-Costa D, Alfonso JF, Montés-Micó R, Poo-López A. Optical and visual performance of diffractive intraocular lens implantation after myopic laser in situ keratomileusis. *J Cataract Refract Surg.* 2009;35(5):825-832.

26
QUESTION

WHAT IS YOUR ROUTINE TESTING FOR PATIENTS WHO ARE RECEIVING A REFRACTIVE IOL?

Preeya K. Gupta, MD and Jay J. Meyer, MD, MPH

Patients receiving a premium or refractive intraocular lens (IOL) (ie, toric, accommodating, or multifocal IOL) have high expectations for final visual outcomes. With this in mind, it behooves the surgeon to perform a thorough preoperative evaluation to exclude or treat any preexisting conditions that may limit best-corrected visual acuity or quality of vision.

The basic goals of the preoperative evaluation include the following:

- Make sure the ocular surface is normal (eg, no dry eye, anterior basement membrane dystrophy, or Salzmann nodules).
- Make sure biometry and IOL calculation formulas are as accurate as possible.
- Have a plan for residual or anticipated astigmatism.
- After reviewing the above, make sure postoperative expectations can be met.

Examination

The preoperative exam includes a detailed evaluation of the ocular surface and fundus, as well as an assessment of the patient's visual goals. Any factors that may influence the patient's outcome should be identified, explained to the patient and, if possible, treated prior to surgery. The most commonly found conditions that impair vision quality include dry eyes, blepharitis, epithelial basement membrane dystrophy, epiretinal membrane, and macular degeneration. Any preexisting condition that is not brought to the patient's attention until after surgery can leave patients with the impression that surgery caused the abnormality or that surgery was a failure because he or she did not achieve his or her expected visual outcome.

Henderson BA, Yoo SH. *Curbside Consultation in Refractive and Lens-Based Surgery: 49 Clinical Questions* (pp 99-102)
© 2015 SLACK Incorporated

The preoperative discussion should elicit the patient's goals and expectations and these should be aligned with the anticipated results. It is important to discuss limitations of IOL calculations, especially with patients that have undergone prior refractive surgery or have extremes of axial length, and also make patients aware of how this can affect their goal of spectacle independence. Similarly, for patients with anticipated residual refractive error or astigmatism, a preliminary plan should be formulated to treat this and discussed with the patient in advance.

Preoperative Testing

There are a number of preoperative tests that can provide the surgeon with more detailed information about the patient's eye. In our practice, the following tests are performed on every refractive IOL patient: manual keratometry, corneal topography, biometry, and optical coherence tomography (OCT).

MANUAL KERATOMETRY AND CORNEAL TOPOGRAPHY

Manual keratometry is useful for evaluating the tear film and providing an additional measurement of astigmatism axis and magnitude. These measurements are compared with topography and automated keratometry measurements of astigmatism. Although there is often a slight variation in magnitude of astigmatism, it is most important to find consistency in the axis of astigmatism between each modality. When there is significant variation, one should be suspicious of an ocular surface abnormality (eg, dry eyes or anterior basement membrane dystrophy).

Corneal topography is used to also evaluate the type and degree of astigmatism. For patients receiving a toric IOL, topography is essential to verify that the astigmatism is regular, and that the axis of astigmatism correlates with keratometry. Topography can also provide clues to ocular surface or corneal issues, as well as irregular astigmatism from keratoconus (inferior steepening), dryness (missing superior data), contact lens warpage (Figure 26-1), and scarring.

BIOMETRY

Accurate biometry is imperative to ensuring the best possible refractive outcomes. An optical biometer such as the Lenstar (Haag-Streit) or the IOLMaster (Carl Zeiss Meditec) is preferred for the average patient given the ease of use (noncontact) and repeatability of measurements. We prefer to have biometry measurements taken prior to the patient receiving any eye drops or applanation to allow the ocular surface to be as undisturbed as possible to achieve the most accurate keratometry values. Attention must be given to the ocular surface because dryness or corneal warpage can affect measurements, especially keratometry values and axis. If evidence of dryness is seen on exam or irregular astigmatism on topography, consider treating the ocular surface and repeating measurements at a later date. When there is difficulty in obtaining measurements due to the ocular surface, the patient can be instructed to blink several times prior to measurements. Application of artificial tears can also be used when there is difficulty obtaining measurements; however, we recommend using a low viscosity artificial tear and waiting at least 5 minutes prior to repeating measurements because viscous artificial tears can cause greater alterations in the tear film[1] that may decrease the accuracy of measurements. For patients wearing contact lenses, we recommend they stay out of their lenses for at least 2 weeks prior to obtaining measurements, as we have seen changes in the predicted lens power calculation of up to 1 diopter (D) on repeat measurements after discontinuing contact lenses (more typical with hard contact lenses). We follow the general rule of thumb: discontinue soft contact lenses for 2 weeks, or 1 week for each decade of rigid gas permeable (RGP) lens use. Even longer intervals may be required for some patients to ensure biometry measurements are stable.

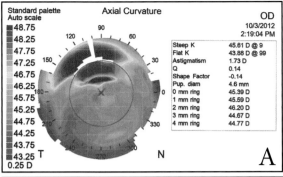

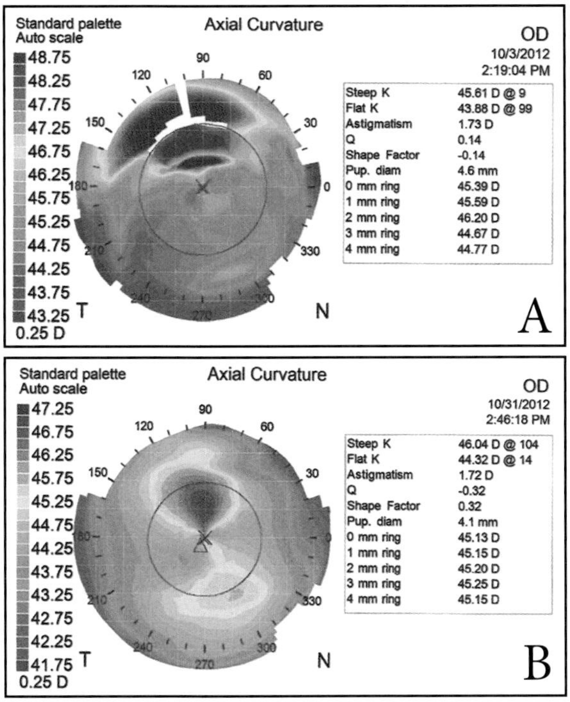

Figure 26-1. (A) Corneal topography showing irregular astigmatism in a contact lens wearer evaluated for toric lens placement. (B) Repeat topography after a 4-week contact lens hiatus showed regular astigmatism with significant change in the steep axis.

Figure 26-2. Lenstar data sheet showing a high flat K and axis measurement standard deviation.

Flat meridian	K1	⚠ 44.81 D @ 67°	±0.491 D
Steep meridian	K2	⚠ 48.03 D @ 157°	±0.156 D
Astigmatism	AST	3.23 D @ 157°	±8.7°
Keratometric index	n	1.3375	

Figure 26-3. Missing data points (X) and variability in the listed IOLMaster keratometry measurements seen in a patient with dry eyes.

MV: 43.95/44.94 D	SD: 0.02 mm		
K1: 43.83 D x 130°	7.70 mm		
K2: 45.12 D x 40°	7.48 mm		
ΔK: +1.29 D x 40°			
K1: 44.18 D x 112°	7.64 mm		O O
K2: 44.47 D x 22°	7.59 mm	O	O
ΔK: +0.29 D x 22°			X O
K1: 43.89 D x 143°	7.69 mm		O O
K2: 45.18 D x 53°	7.47 mm	O	O
ΔK: +1.29 D x 53°			X O

Another clue suggesting imprecision of measurements is a high standard deviation (SD). We recommend inspecting the data sheet portion of the IOL calculations to identify any variability in measurements. Keratometry measurements should be repeated if the SD is greater than 0.25 D or if axis SD is greater than 3.5 degrees when using the Lenstar for a toric lens (Figure 26-2).[2] The Lenstar also allows the operator to review and exclude outliers from the calculations. When using the IOLMaster, missing keratometry data points or variability in the listed measurements suggests the need to repeat measurements and examine the ocular surface (Figure 26-3).

It is recommended that surgeons track their refractive outcomes and optimize their A-constants for the best possible IOL calculations, with preference given to later-generation formulas. For patients who have undergone prior refractive surgery, we recommend reviewing old refractive surgery records when available and using the ASCRS calculator (http://iolcalc.org) to determine the adjusted IOL power.

Optical Coherence Tomography

For patients with known macular disease, OCT can define the extent of disease to provide prognostic information that guides preoperative counseling and treatment decisions. A macular OCT is also invaluable as a screening tool for the identification of subtle macular pathology that could be missed on dilated fundus examination. This includes macular edema, epiretinal membranes,[3] macular holes, and vitreomacular traction. In cases of suspected pathology or when symptoms are out of proportion to any anterior segment pathology, it is especially important to scroll through the images to verify that there is no pathology throughout the entire imaged macula rather than relying on one single horizontal image/slice through the central fovea.

Conclusion

Identification of preexisting conditions that could lead to suboptimal refractive outcomes is paramount when assessing a candidate for a refractive IOL. Special attention should be paid to the ocular surface, corneal topography, biometry, and OCT.

References

1. Wang J, Simmons P, Aquavella J, et al. Dynamic distribution of artificial tears on the ocular surface. *Arch Ophthalmol.* 2008;126(5):619-625.
2. http://www.haag-streit-usa.com/mylenstar/lenstar-videos/training.aspx. Accessed January 6, 2013.
3. Milani P, Raimondi G, Morale D, Scialdone A. Biomicroscopy versus optical coherence tomography screening of epiretinal membranes in patients undergoing cataract surgery. *Retina.* 2012;32(5):897-904.

SECTION V

ASTIGMATISM CORRECTION

WHAT IS YOUR ALGORITHM FOR CHOOSING WHEN TO PERFORM A CORNEAL INCISIONAL ASTIGMATIC CORRECTION VS TORIC IOL VS LASER REFRACTIVE SURGERY?

Francesco Carones, MD

The recent developments in cataract surgery, such as presbyopia-correcting intraocular lenses (IOLs), as well as the greater patient expectations and requests, highlight the need to obtain perfect outcomes with plano refraction after the surgical procedure. Certainly, preexisting astigmatism is one challenge the surgeon has to manage properly to reach this goal.

There may be different approaches to correct astigmatism, either simultaneously with the cataract procedure, or at a later stage.[1] In order to properly manage it, it is very important to have a clear understanding of the characteristics of preexisting astigmatism, and of the systematic astigmatism that is induced with the surgical technique.

The assessment of preexisting astigmatism may be done with different diagnostics. My approach involves corneal topography performed with two different devices (to screen for regularity and precise axis determination, and to measure anterior corneal curvature toricity), optical coherence biometry performed with two different devices (useful to measure K-readings and axis determination), and Scheimpflug camera tomography (to assess posterior corneal curvature toricity, to be added to/subtracted from the anterior one). I don't perform manual keratometry any longer. I am using different devices in order to check for consistency of the measurements.

There are different scenarios based on the results of the preoperative assessment. The ideal condition is when the amount of measured astigmatism is consistent among the different instrument measurements, and corneal topography shows a regular, symmetric bowtie pattern with no irregularity generated by tear film alteration (Figure 27-1). In these cases, I prefer to correct astigmatism using toric IOLs. In my hands, this approach is more precise, faster, more reliable, and better accepted by the patients.[2] I prefer to implant a toric IOL in cases where the resulting astigmatism measured by diagnostics is 0.75 diopters (D) or greater; this number reduces to

Henderson BA, Yoo SH. *Curbside Consultation in Refractive
and Lens-Based Surgery: 49 Clinical Questions* (pp 105-107)
© 2015 SLACK Incorporated

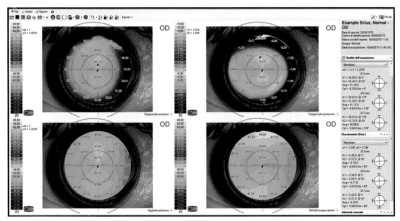

Figure 27-1. This quad image taken with a Scheimpflug camera presents the ideal condition for correcting astigmatism with a toric IOL. The anterior surface tangential and axial maps (top and bottom left) show a regular, symmetric bowtie pattern. The posterior surface tangential map (top right) shows the same regular pattern. The refractive-equivalent map (bottom right) displays the total amount of astigmatism by subtracting the posterior surface toricity from the anterior surface one, being the posterior surface negative values.

0.50 D when implanting a multifocal IOL. I don't make the incision on the steeper meridian as part of my routine surgery. I implant the IOL through a 2-mm incision in almost all cases, setting the incision on the temporal side. I learned that my average induced astigmatism is 0.15 D with a very small standard deviation, and this is the number I consider for calculating the amount of astigmatism to be corrected with the IOL. My target is getting as close to plano as possible, but avoiding overcorrection.

In my hands and according to literature, incisional surgery to correct astigmatism is less accurate and precise than toric IOLs.[3] Most of my patients don't like the idea of having additional cuts on the eye, and I don't like the fluctuation and the long-term changes resulting from the correction of astigmatism through an incision. This is why I prefer to correct preexisting astigmatism with the IOL. However, when the preoperative assessment is not ideal, I prefer to correct astigmatism with incisions at the time of surgery. This is especially the case in irregular astigmatism with skewed axis (nonorthogonal semimeridians at corneal topography [Figure 27-2]) and asymmetric astigmatism (asymmetric bowtie pattern at corneal topography [Figure 27-3]), where an IOL cannot correct the irregularity and/or the asymmetry. I therefore implant a standard monofocal IOL and perform incisional surgery. However, when the difference between steeper and flatter axis is significant, or the amount of astigmatism to correct is greater than 1.5 D, I prefer not to correct it at the time of surgery but at a later stage because of the difficulty in correcting it. Once the cataract has been removed, it is easier to assess the impact of these kinds of irregular/asymmetric astigmatism on best-corrected visual acuity, and have a better understanding of the refractive implications. Wavefront analysis and corneal topography at this stage are very helpful, and for most of these uncommon cases the best treatment is a corneal wavefront-guided excimer laser procedure, which compensates for corneal irregularity and asymmetry.

As in the previous situation, astigmatism correction with a second-step surgical procedure after cataract surgery comes as a planned approach in only a few specific cases. In all these cases, I prefer the excimer laser to incisional surgery because of the more accurate and reliable results, and the greater patient acceptance. Most of these cases can be easily treated by surface ablation, which I think is the procedure of choice in the elderly because these patients very often have tear film issues. For those more demanding patients, femtosecond laser–assisted LASIK can also be considered, but I

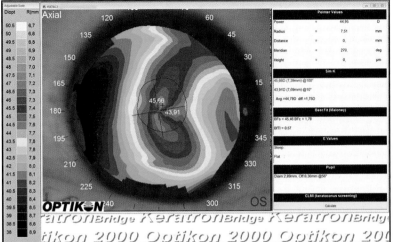

Figure 27-2. This anterior surface corneal topography shows astigmatism with skewed, non-orthogonal axes. In these cases, I prefer to use incisional surgery to correct astigmatism because of the inability of toric IOLs to correct astigmatism resulting from nonorthogonal axes. Incisions are to be placed on the 60- and 300-degree semimeridians.

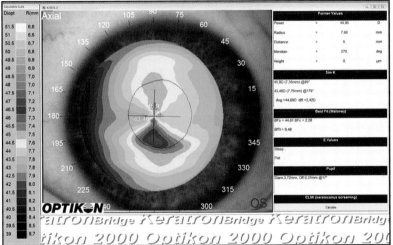

Figure 27-3. This anterior surface corneal topography presents an asymmetric bowtie pattern where the lower semimeridian is steeper than the upper one. In these cases, toric IOLs cannot fully correct the astigmatism resulting from asymmetry. I correct these cases by placing asymmetric incisions in length on the same meridian.

perform it only when the tear film is very stable to avoid dry eye symptoms and long recovery times. I like to plan correction of astigmatism with a second surgical step in cases with very long or very short eyes, as well as high astigmatic eyes for which my preferred aspheric standard or multifocal toric IOL is not available in power. I tend to leave as low refractive error as possible after the implant (for both sphere and cylinder), to be fine-tuned with the excimer laser 2 to 3 months after cataract surgery.

References

1. Rubenstein JB, Raciti M. Approaches to corneal astigmatism in cataract surgery. *Curr Opin Ophthalmol.* 2013;24(1):30-34.
2. Poll JT, Wang L, Koch DD, Weikert MP. Correction of astigmatism during cataract surgery: Toric intraocular lens compared to peripheral corneal relaxing incisions. *J Refract Surg.* 2011;27(3):165-171.
3. Mingo-Botín D, Muñoz-Negrete FJ, Won Kim HR, Morcillo-Laiz R, Rebolleda G, Oblanca N. Comparison of toric intraocular lenses and peripheral corneal relaxing incisions to treat astigmatism during cataract surgery. *J Cataract Refract Surg.* 2010;36(10):1700-1708.

28

CAN I USE A TORIC IOL IN A PATIENT WITH KERATOCONUS? HOW ABOUT IN A PATIENT WITH EBMD, FUCHS', OR OTHER CORNEAL DYSTROPHIES?

Mahshad Darvish-Zargar, MD CM, MBA, FRCSC
and Edward J. Holland, MD

Since their introduction, toric intraocular lenses (IOLs) have become an important tool to help ophthalmologists achieve the best possible refractive results. Initially, surgeons were only using these lenses in patients with no other anterior segment pathology. With time and experience, we are seeing that toric IOLs can play an expanded role and be used in various corneal pathologies.

Keratoconus

Keratoconus is a progressive disease characterized by thinning and ectasia of the cornea. This often results in large amounts of irregular astigmatism and myopia. Although the onset is generally at puberty, progression can occur into the third and fourth decades of life. These patients also develop visually significant cataracts at a younger age compared with the general population.

The treatment of keratoconus is dependent on the severity of the disease. Mild and moderate cases can be treated with spectacles and rigid gas-permeable contact lenses. More advanced cases may require surgery, including intracorneal ring segments and anterior lamellar or penetrating keratoplasty. Recently, mild and moderate cases are also being treated with corneal collagen cross-linking using riboflavin and ultraviolet light. The goal of this therapy is to stop the progression of the disease and avoid future surgical interventions.

We believe that toric IOLs are a valid therapeutic option for appropriate patients. Just as with any other keratoconic patients, these patients should have regular topography and manifest refractions. If the patient has had a previous penetrating or anterior lamellar keratoplasty, we do not advocate the use of toric IOLs. The reason for this is that should this patient's transplant fail,

Henderson BA, Yoo SH. *Curbside Consultation in Refractive and Lens-Based Surgery: 49 Clinical Questions* (pp 109-111)
© 2015 SLACK Incorporated

he or she would have two sources of toricity: the new transplant and the toric IOL, leading to a potentially difficult situation to correct using contact lenses, spectacles, or surface ablation.

The ideal patient for a toric IOL would be a patient who has not had a previous keratoplasty, has had stable topography and astigmatism for at least 1 year, and is in at least the fourth decade of life. Patients who have a significant visual improvement with a manifest refraction are expected to have the best outcomes. There have been several papers exploring the use of toric IOLs and they have had positive results, significantly reducing postoperative cylinder and improving uncorrected visual acuity up to 1 year postoperatively.[1-3]

The final refractive outcomes are more variable than standard cases due to several factors. First, the preoperative measurements are more difficult due to the irregular corneal astigmatism and steep Ks. The surgically induced astigmatism has also been described as less predictable and highly variable, likely due to the altered biomechanical properties of the cornea.[4] Lastly, the range of the toric multifocal lenses limits the reductions in final refractive astigmatism.

Overall, we feel that cataract extraction with toric IOL implantation is a good surgical intervention to reduce the irregular astigmatism of patients who have stable and mild to moderate keratoconus and to achieve optimal visual outcomes.

Epithelial Basement Membrane Degeneration

Epithelial basement membrane degeneration (EBMD) is a common condition that affects the epithelium and anterior cornea, causing the characteristic slit-lamp findings of maps (redundant sheets of basement membrane that extend into the corneal epithelium), dots (epithelial cysts), and fingerprints (thickened basement membrane). These surface irregularities can cause unreliable K readings, leading to difficulties in deciding if the patient would benefit from a toric IOL. Topography will also show an irregular map with areas of dropout. Lastly, EBMD may be one of the factors decreasing the patient's vision, and cataract surgery alone may not fully optimize his or her visual potential.

If you have any concern that the EBMD findings you see on the slit-lamp are affecting the patient's vision or your IOL measurements, we recommend that you perform at least a superficial keratectomy and, if possible, a phototherapeutic keratectomy as well. Once the epithelium is healed and the corneal surface is smooth, you can reevaluate the patient for cataract surgery.

Stromal Dystrophies

We do not recommend the use of a toric IOL for any patient who may need to undergo a penetrating or anterior lamellar corneal transplant or has already undergone one. The explanation for this is the same as that for keratoconus patients that already have or may require a corneal transplant.

Fuchs' Dystrophy

Fuchs' dystrophy involves swelling of the endothelial layer of the cornea, which in turn causes glare, halos, and decreased visual acuity. When considering cataract surgery on these patients, it is important to develop a grading scale for the severity of the condition; this will also help with the decision of using a toric IOL.

We grade our Fuchs' dystrophy patients in the following fashion:

1. Mild guttata: These patients have no real risk of corneal decompensation. If the patient has corneal astigmatism, then a toric IOL can be recommended.

2. Confluent guttata with no evidence of stromal edema: These cases will only require phaco, but the possibility of a future endothelial keratoplasty (EK) must be discussed. A toric lens is an option in these cases; however, patients must be aware that should they require an EK, their refractive status will change.

3. Confluent guttata with possible stromal edema: These patients have a very high risk of requiring an EK in the near future. A toric IOL is not recommended. If there is evidence of morning stromal edema, consider a combined procedure.

4. Confluent guttata with definite edema: For these patients, we recommend a combined cataract extraction and EK. Once again, a toric IOL is not recommended.

These recommendations hold true for both Descemet's stripping endothelial keratoplasty (DSEK) and ultra-thin DSEK because both change the posterior curvature of the cornea and change the refractive status. Descemet's membrane endothelial keratoplasty appears not to change the refractive status of the patient, and therefore toric IOLs may be an option in patients requiring EK in the future.

References

1. Nanavaty MA, Lake DA, Daya SM. Outcomes of pseudophakic toric intraocular lens implantation in keratoconic eyes with cataract. *J Refract Surg.* 2012;28(12):884-889.
2. Jaimes M, Xacur-García F, Alvarez-Melloni D, Graue-Hernández EO, Ramirez-Luquín T, Navas A. Refractive lens exchange with toric intraocular lenses in keratoconus. *J Refract Surg.* 2011;27(9):658-664.
3. Navas A, Suarez R. One-year follow-up of toric intraocular lens implantation in forme fruste keratoconus. *J Cataract Refract Surg.* 2009; 35:2024-2027.
4. Visser N, Gast STJM, Bauer NJC, Nuijts RMMA. Cataract surgery with toric intraocular lens implantation in keratoconus: A case report. *Cornea.* 2011;30:720-723.

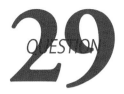

IF THE K MEASUREMENTS DIFFER BETWEEN DIFFERENT METHODS, WHICH ONE SHOULD I USE?

Nienke Visser, MD and Rudy M.M.A. Nuijts, MD, PhD

Accurate corneal astigmatism measurements must be obtained to make sure you achieve success with toric intraocular lenses (IOLs). Many different devices are currently available to measure keratometry (K) values and corresponding meridians. Our preferred method to measure K-values is with the IOLMaster (Carl Zeiss Meditec). In our experience, the automated keratometry feature of the IOLMaster minimizes problems related to human errors. Furthermore, it is a reliable tool in spherical power calculations. In addition, because the IOLMaster always performs 3 repeated keratometry measurements, you can be sure that reliable and repeatable K-value measurements are taken. To measure astigmatism meridians, we compare measurements obtained with the IOLMaster, a corneal topographer, and a manual keratometer. In most patients, the values between the IOLMaster and corneal topographer are consistent with each other within 5 degrees. In these patients, we use the measurements obtained with the IOLMaster. If the discrepancy is more than 5 degrees, you have to be careful. First, you should confirm that measurements obtained with both devices are of good quality, reliable, and that no irregular corneal astigmatism (eg, due to keratoconus) exists. In our clinic, all patients who choose to have a toric IOL undergo manual keratometry using the Javal-Schiøtz keratometer (Rodenstock), which we still regard as the gold standard for meridian determination. In patients with a 5-degree difference between the astigmatism meridians obtained with the IOLMaster and corneal topographer, we usually use the meridians measured with the Javal-Schiøtz keratometer.

Henderson BA, Yoo SH. *Curbside Consultation in Refractive and Lens-Based Surgery: 49 Clinical Questions* (pp 113-115)
© 2015 SLACK Incorporated

Figure 29-1. Light reflections projected by the (A) IOLMaster, (B) Lenstar, and (C) Javal-Schiøtz manual keratometer onto the cornea to measure the anterior curvature.

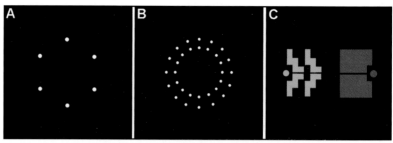

Why Do K Measurements Differ Between Different Methods?

Most devices calculate keratometry values based on the curvature of the anterior cornea. Several methods are available to measure the curvature of the anterior cornea. For example, the IOLMaster projects six spots of light in a hexagonal pattern on the anterior cornea and uses the reflections to determine the anterior radius of curvature (Figure 29-1A). The Lenstar (Haag-Streit) uses the same technique but projects 32 lights, divided into 2 rings, onto the cornea (Figure 29-1B). Corneal topographers use Placido-disc videokeratoscopy using the optical reflections of 19 illuminated rings. The Javal-Schiøtz keratometer requires subjective alignment of 2 keratometer mires (a red square and green staircase) along the principal meridians of the cornea (Figure 29-1C). We found that corneal topographers showed the best repeatability when measuring K-values. This is to be expected because Placido-disc corneal topographers gather more data points compared with other keratometers. However, the repeatability in measuring the astigmatism meridian was comparable for all devices (a standard deviation of 21 to 26 degrees for 3 repeatable measurements). We believe that this is too high in cases of toric IOL implantation. We recommend that before calculating a toric IOL cylinder power and alignment axis, a series of repeatable astigmatism measurements must be obtained to ensure repeatable meridian measurements.

Another source for differences between keratometers is that different devices measure different zones of the cornea. For example, the IOLMaster and Lenstar use a central 2.3-mm zone, corneal topographers generally use a 3.0-mm zone, and manual keratometry uses a 3.4-mm zone. Because the normal cornea is aspheric, the central cornea is steeper than the peripheral cornea. However, in our experience, differences in K-values between devices are small (approximately 0.12 diopters [D] or less) and therefore not clinically relevant.[1]

Also, different refractive indices may be used to calculate the corneal power (D) from the radius of curvature (mm). Most devices use a refractive index of 1.3375 (IOLMaster, corneal topography), although some devices use a refractive index of 1.3320 (Lenstar). When you compare K-values obtained with different devices for the same patient, make sure that the refractive indices are the same. For example, an anterior radius of curvature of 7.50 mm results in a corneal power of 45.0 D using an index of 1.3375, or 44.3 D using an index of 1.3320. However, differences are small when calculating the absolute astigmatism values.

Another technique to measure keratometry or corneal power is based on both the anterior and posterior cornea surface. Whereas the aforementioned techniques determine the corneal curvature using reflections on the tear film, these techniques only measure the anterior surface of the cornea. A rotating Scheimpflug camera (Pentacam) measures both the anterior and posterior corneal curvature and uses the correct refractive indices for cornea and aqueous. However, corneal powers based on these parameters are significantly different from keratometry measurements.[1,2] Even though these Pentacam parameters cannot be used in conventional IOL calculation formulas, the posterior cornea may be considered in toric IOL calculations. As recently shown by Koch, the posterior corneal surface acts as a minus lens and affects corneal astigmatism.[3] Ignoring posterior corneal astigmatism leads to overcorrection in with-the-rule astigmatism, and undercorrection in eyes with against-the-rule astigmatism.[3]

References

1. Visser N, Berendschot TTJM, Verbakel F, Brabander de J, Nuijts RMMA. Comparability and repeatability of corneal astigmatism measurements using different measurement technologies. *J Cataract Refract Surg.* 2012;38:1764-1770.
2. Symes RJ, Ursell PG. Automated keratometry in routine cataract surgery: Comparison of Scheimpflug and conventional values. *J Cataract Refract Surg.* 2011;37:295-301.
3. Koch DD, Ali SF, Weikert MP, Shirayama M, Jenkins R, Wang L. Contribution of posterior corneal astigmatism to total corneal astigmatism. *J Cataract Refract Surg.* 2012;38:2080-2087.

QUESTION 30

IS POSTERIOR CORNEAL ASTIGMATISM IMPORTANT WHEN PLANNING CATARACT SURGERY?

Zaina Al-Mohtaseb, MD; Bruna V. Ventura, MD, MS; Li Wang, MD, PhD; and Douglas D. Koch, MD

Accurate assessment of the total corneal refractive power is vital for calculating intraocular lens (IOL) power and managing corneal astigmatism during cataract surgery. Traditionally, the magnitude of the posterior corneal astigmatism has been considered clinically negligible because of the small difference in refractive indices between the cornea and the aqueous.[1] Thus, keratometry or computerized videokeratography (CVK) have been used to directly measure the anterior corneal surface and to estimate the refractive power of the total cornea using a standardized index of refraction.[2] However, in many cases, this results in significant residual astigmatism after surgery.[3]

Our interest in this topic evolved from noting unexpected toric IOL outcomes in our practice. For example, a 71-year-old female presented for preoperative evaluation for cataract surgery. In the left eye, the corrected distance visual acuity (CDVA) was 20/40 and the manifest refraction was –5.75 +2.50 X 176. The measured corneal astigmatism was 0.95 diopters (D) @ 169 with the Atlas corneal topography (Carl Zeiss Meditec), 1.34 D @ 176 with the IOLMaster device (Carl Zeiss Meditec AG), and 1.64 D @ 173 with the Lenstar device (Haag-Streit AG). An Alcon SN6AT4 was implanted for near vision to correct for 1.50 D of corneal astigmatism at 175 degrees. One month postoperatively, the uncorrected distance visual acuity (UDVA) was 20/60, the manifest refraction was –2.25 +1.00 X 165, and the corneal astigmatism was undercorrected by 1 D. Concurrently with these clinical observations, we had begun using Scheimpflug imaging, which can measure the posterior corneal curvature, to investigate the contribution of posterior corneal astigmatism to overall corneal astigmatism and to calculate the error introduced by estimating the total corneal astigmatism from only the anterior corneal measurements.

Using the Galilei Dual Scheimpflug Analyzer (Ziemer Ophthalmic Systems AG), we measured the corneas of 715 eyes of 434 patients, with ages ranging from 20 to 80 years.[4] We compared corneal astigmatism derived from the total corneal power displayed on the device, which accounts

Henderson BA, Yoo SH. *Curbside Consultation in Refractive and Lens-Based Surgery: 49 Clinical Questions* (pp 117-120)
© 2015 SLACK Incorporated

for the contributions of the anterior and posterior corneal surfaces, with the corneal astigmatism from simulated keratometry (CA_{SimK}), which is based only on anterior corneal measurements. We then calculated the estimation error for CA_{SimK}, which is the error introduced by calculating total corneal astigmatism based only on anterior surface measurements.

We found a mean estimation error of 0.22 D @ 180, with 5% of eyes having an error greater than 0.50 D. In addition, the mean magnitude of posterior corneal astigmatism, which was directly measured by the Galilei, was –0.30 D and 9% of eyes had more than 0.50 D of posterior corneal astigmatism. Strikingly, the posterior corneal surface was steepest vertically in 86.6% of corneas. Interestingly, with increasing age, the steep anterior corneal meridian shifts from with-the-rule (WTR) to against-the-rule (ATR), whereas the posterior corneal steep meridian was steep vertically in the majority of corneas in all age groups.

Because the posterior corneal surface acts as a minus lens, a steeper curvature at the 90-degree meridian creates net plus refractive power horizontally. Thus, posterior corneal astigmatism partially compensates for anterior corneal astigmatism in corneas that have WTR astigmatism on the anterior corneal surface, but increases total corneal astigmatism in corneas that have ATR anterior corneal astigmatism.

The magnitude of posterior corneal astigmatism varies according to the anterior corneal astigmatism. In corneas having WTR astigmatism on the anterior surface, mean posterior corneal astigmatism is approximately 0.5 D, and the magnitude increases as the anterior astigmatism increases, partially compensating for the anterior increase. Conversely, in the ATR eyes, mean posterior astigmatism is approximately 0.3 D and is not correlated with anterior values. The clinical impact is that, if we base our astigmatic corrections on anterior corneal measurements only, there will be a tendency to overcorrect WTR corneas and undercorrect ATR corneas.

As a result of these findings, we developed a new nomogram to guide the selection of toric IOLs, and we changed our existing nomogram for peripheral corneal relaxing incisions (PCRIs) (Tables 30-1 to 30-4). Recently, a 71-year-old female presented for preoperative evaluation for cataract surgery. In the left eye, the CDVA was 20/40 and the manifest refraction was –13.00 +2.00 X 75. The measured corneal astigmatism was 2.50 D @ 84 with Atlas corneal topography, 2.07 D @ 88 with the IOLMaster device, and 2.00 D @ 85 with the Lenstar device. In the past, we would have implanted a SN6AT5 lens, but, as a result of our recent research, an Alcon SN6AT4 was implanted for intermediate vision to correct for 1.50 D of corneal astigmatism @ 88. One month postoperatively, the UDVA was 20/40 and the manifest refraction was –1.00 +0.25 X 80.

The ultimate goal of the ongoing studies is evolution of current devices and development of new ones that will enable us to accurately measure total corneal astigmatism and power, solving this problem and others, such as accuracy of spherical IOL power calculations in eyes that have undergone corneal refractive surgery.

References

1. Cheng L, Tsai C, Tsai RJ, Liou S, Ho J. Estimation accuracy of surgically induced astigmatism on the cornea when neglecting the posterior corneal surface measurement. *Acta Ophthalmol*. 2011; 89:417-422.
2. Wang L, Mahmoud A, Anderson B, Koch D, Roberts C. Total corneal power estimation: Ray tracing method versus gaussian optics formula. *Invest Ophthalmol Vis Sci*. 2011;52(3):1716-1722.
3. Mendicute J, Irigoyen C, Aramberri J, Ondarra A, Montes-Mico R. Foldable toric intraocular lens for astigmatism correction in cataract patients. *J Cataract Refract Surg*. 2008;34:601-607.
4. Koch D, Ali S, Weikert MP, Shirayama M, Jenkins R, Wang L. Contribution of posterior corneal astigmatism to total corneal astigmatism. *J Cataract Refract Surg*. 2012;38(12):2080-2087.

Table 30-1

Baylor Toric IOL Nomogram for the Alcon SN6ATT Lens

Toric IOL	WTR, D	ATR, D
0	≤1.69 (PCRI if > 1.00)	≤0.39
T3 (1.03*)	1.70 to 2.19	0.40** to 0.79
T4 (1.55*)	2.20 to 2.69	0.80 to 1.29
T5 (2.06*)	2.70 to 3.19	1.30 to 1.79
T6 (2.57*)	3.20 to 3.69	1.80 to 2.29
T7 (3.08*)	3.70 to 4.19	2.30 to 2.79
T8 (3.60*)	4.20 to 4.69	2.80 to 3.29
T9 (4.11*)	4.70 to 5.19	3.30 to 3.79

Values are the vector sum of the anterior corneal and surgically induced astigmatisms.
Abbreviations: ATR, against-the-rule; PCRI, peripheral corneal-relaxing incision; WTR, with-the-rule.
*Effective IOL cylinder power at corneal plane.
**Especially if spectacles have more ATR.

Table 30-2

Baylor Toric IOL Nomogram for the AMO ZCT Lens

Toric IOL	WTR, D	ATR, D
0	≤1.69 (PCRI if > 1.00)	≤0.39
ZCT150 (1.03*)	1.70 to 2.19	0.40** to 0.79
ZCT225 (1.55*)	2.20 to 2.69	0.80 to 1.29
ZCT300 (2.06*)	2.70 to 3.24	1.30 to 1.79
ZCT400 (2.74*)	3.25 to 4.00	1.80 to 2.50

Values are the vector sum of the anterior corneal and surgically induced astigmatisms.
Abbreviations: ATR, against-the-rule; PCRI, peripheral corneal-relaxing incision; WTR, with-the-rule.
*Effective IOL cylinder power at corneal plane.
**Especially if spectacles have more ATR.

Table 30-3

PCRI Nomogram for With-the-Rule Astigmatism and a 2.4-mm Temporal Clear Corneal Incision

Preoperative Astigmatism, D	Age, y	Number	Length, degrees
1.25 to 1.75	<65	2	35*
	≥65	1	35
>1.75	<65	2	60
	≥65	2	45

Abbreviation: PCRI, peripheral corneal-relaxing incision.
*Or 1 PCRI of 50 degrees if asymmetric astigmatism.

Table 30-4

PCRI Nomogram for Against-the-Rule or Oblique Astigmatism and a 2.4-mm Temporal Clear Corneal Incision

Preoperative Astigmatism, D	Age, y	Number	Length, degrees
0.4 to 0.8	-	1	35 to 40*
0.81 to 1.2	-	1	45
	-	2	40
≥1.2	-	2	45

Abbreviation: PCRI, peripheral corneal-relaxing incision.
*Or paired PCRIs of 30 degrees if symmetric astigmatism.
For against-the-rule astigmatism, consider doing PCRIs especially if a clear corneal incision is not centered with corneal astigmatism.

HOW DO I DETERMINE
MY SURGICALLY INDUCED ASTIGMATISM?

Alex Mammen, MD and Deepinder K. Dhaliwal, MD, LAc

An understanding of one's aggregate surgically induced astigmatism (SIA) helps in the quest for refractive predictability after cataract surgery. Free online calculators simplify the calculations involved in this vector analysis, but require reliable input data to yield accurate and meaningful results.

As cataract surgery has become increasingly refined, both the desire and achievability of spectacle independence have correspondingly increased. Hitting the target refraction cannot be reliably achieved, however, without a quantitative understanding of the astigmatism that is induced by the surgical incision.

The definition of SIA is the difference between postoperative and preoperative corneal astigmatism. However, because astigmatism is a vector quantity with both magnitude (power) and direction (axis), this difference is not just a matter of simple subtraction. Rather, geometric vector analysis or a trigonometric conversion of vectors into mathematical equations is necessary. There have been various methods published with varying levels of ease and efficacy.[1] Fortunately, you do not have to worry about brushing up on your mathematical skills due to the availability of free online programs that will perform the calculations for you (www.doctor-hill.com/physicians/sia_calculator.htm or www.insighteyeclinic.in/SIA_calculator.php).

The integrity of these calculations, of course, depends on the quality of the data entered. The measurement of preoperative and postoperative astigmatism should be accurate and stable. Commonly used methods to measure astigmatism include manual keratometry, optical biometry with the Haag-Streit Lenstar or Zeiss IOLMaster, autokeratometry, and topography. We rely more heavily on manual keratometry and Lenstar measurements in our practice. Preoperatively, stability is mainly influenced by contact lens wear. Similar to refractive surgery guidelines, soft nontoric contact lens wearers should ideally stay out of their contacts for 2 weeks, with a 3-week

Henderson BA, Yoo SH. *Curbside Consultation in Refractive*
and Lens-Based Surgery: 49 Clinical Questions (pp 121-122)
© 2015 SLACK Incorporated

holiday recommended for toric and hard contact lens wearers. If possible, stability should be confirmed with repeat measurements at least 1 week apart. Similar stability should be confirmed postoperatively, with measurements usually taken between 4 to 6 weeks after surgery, after all corneal sutures have been removed. The same method/instrument should be used to perform the pre- and postoperative measurement of astigmatism.

While the magnitude of SIA varies by surgeon, incision size, and location, the average for temporal clear corneal incisions is approximately 0.5 to 0.6 diopters (D).[2,3] It generally takes at least 20 uniform, uncomplicated cases to yield a reliable result.[2] Cases should be similar in the following incision characteristics: type (scleral, limbal, or corneal), length, and location (superior, temporal, or other axis). Other subtle factors that can introduce variability are stretching of the incision during surgery and length of the tunnel, with shorter tunnels causing more flattening.

While the aforementioned online calculators can be utilized to measure the SIA for a single case, the greater utility is for aggregate analysis to apply toward future surgical planning. Of the two online calculators previously listed, Dr. Warren Hill's provides you with a quantitative SIA result that can either stand alone or be coupled with the online Alcon Acrysof toric IOL calculator (www.acrysoftoriccalculator.com). The calculator from the Insight Eye Clinic can also help predict an estimated postoperative corneal astigmatism for your future nontoric cases. Putting in the work toward understanding your induced corneal astigmatism can help you optimize your cataract surgery results.

References

1. Holladay JT, Cravy TV, Koch DD. Calculating the surgically induced refractive change following ocular surgery. *J Cataract Refract Surg.* 1992;18:429-443.
2. Ernest P, Hill W, Potvin R. Minimizing surgically induced astigmatism at the time of cataract surgery using a square posterior limbal incision. *J Ophthalmol.* 2011;2011:243170.
3. Klamann MK, Gonnermann J, Maier AK, Torun N, Bertelmann E. Smaller incision size leads to higher predictability in microcoaxial cataract surgery. *Eur J Ophthalmol.* 2013;23(2):202-207.

WHAT IS THE BEST WAY TO
MARK THE EYE FOR A TORIC IOL?

Kevin M. Miller, MD

The goal of toric intraocular lens (IOL) implantation is to neutralize postoperative corneal cylinder and thereby eliminate postoperative manifest astigmatism. It is achieved by aligning the axis of the correcting plus cylinder with the meridian of steepest postoperative corneal astigmatism.

Although simple in concept, there are many potential sources of error as this is being done. Inaccuracies may be introduced while (1) positioning a patient's head at the corneal topographer, (2) establishing the limbal reference mark, (3) marking the steep corneal meridian, (4) predicting the surgically induced astigmatism, and (5) aligning the toric IOL with the steep corneal meridian. Inaccuracies in predicting surgically induced astigmatism may arise from two sources: placing the phacoemulsification incision away from the intended corneal meridian, and not obtaining the desired relaxing effect from it. Fortunately, these errors usually do not sum in an absolute value sense.

My current method of marking the eye for toric IOL implantation has evolved over the years to address at least some of these problems.

Current Method

It is important to obtain accurate keratometry readings, but not from a keratometer. The instrument should look at the entire cornea, not just the 3-mm optical zone. Significant variations in corneal power and meridian can be found across an entrance pupil. Eyes with significant irregular astigmatism, such as those with keratoconus, may not be good candidates for toric lens implantation. It is essential, therefore, to use corneal topography or a topography-derived image from a Scheimpflug camera. For my calculations, I use simulated keratometry readings from the 3-mm optical zone of a Pentacam sagittal power map (Oculus USA).

Henderson BA, Yoo SH. *Curbside Consultation in Refractive and Lens-Based Surgery: 49 Clinical Questions* (pp 123-127)
© 2015 SLACK Incorporated

Figure 32-1. A reference mark is made at the 6 o'clock limbus using a fine tip marking pen.

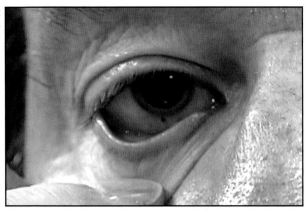

The greatest inaccuracy introduced at this step is head tilt. It is possible to introduce a corneal steep meridian error by tilting a patient's head to the left or right. It does not take much to get a 5- or 10-degree error. It is important that a patient's head be perfectly vertical when the topography map is obtained.

The next step is to place a reference mark on the limbus when the patient is in the operating room. I use an operating table that folds into a chair. I sit the patient perfectly upright and adjust the chair so that the patient's head and mine are at the same height. I then cover the eye that is not undergoing surgery with my hand and make a reference mark at the 6 o'clock limbus using the fine tip end of a Kendall Devon dual tip skin marker (Covidien). I instruct the patient to look at my eye while I make this mark. Errors can be introduced at this step if the patient's head is tilted to either side or if it is extended backward. Care must be exercised to keep the patient's head perfectly vertical, just as when obtaining the topography map. Errors can also be introduced if the spot made by the felt tip marker spreads or "bleeds" after contact with the eye. It's important to use a marker with a fine tip. The limbus should be dry at the point of contact. I find it easier to make a single reference mark at 6 o'clock rather than two reference marks at 3 and 9 o'clock. Only one spot is necessary to establish a rotational reference (Figure 32-1).

The next step is to mark the steep meridian of postoperative corneal cylinder under the operating microscope. A toric calculator is used to determine this meridian preoperatively. At this step, I use an Epsilon ET-04 (Epsilon USA) toric marker. I like this particular marker because it has a low profile, so that the axis numbers on the marker and the eye itself are in focus at the same time. The Epsilon marker has a small diameter so that the entire limbus can be seen while it is being applied. It can be used in eyes that are deep set or have narrow lid fissures. The two blades on the underside of the toric marker are inked with the fat tip side of the Kendall Devon marker. The steep meridian is dialed in according to the results of the toric calculator. The 90-degree meridian on the toric marker is aligned with the reference mark at the 6 o'clock limbus (Figure 32-2).

Before pressing the toric marker onto the cornea, the eye must be completely dry. I do not wet the cornea for 1 or 2 minutes prior to making the toric marks. I use Weck-Cel sponges (Beaver-Visitec International) to soak up any fluid in the cul-de-sac. Once the cornea is dry, I press the toric mark onto it and lift. I try to be perfectly centered over the cornea when I press it down. I then dot the limbus on both sides. The corneal marks will fade as surgery proceeds, but the limbal marks will last throughout the case. When I place the two steep-axis limbal marks, I take the opportunity to correct for any centration errors that I made when pressing the toric marker onto the cornea (Figure 32-3).

The last step is aligning the marks on the toric IOL to the limbal marks at the steep meridian. It is important for the surgeon to avoid leaving any viscoelastic material inside the eye. Doing so might cause the IOL to rotate postoperatively.

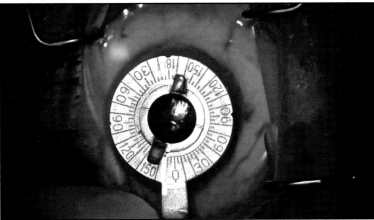

Figure 32-2. A toric marker is pressed against the cornea. The 90-degree meridian on the toric marker aligns with the 6 o'clock limbal reference. The steep postoperative corneal meridian will be 70 degrees in this example.

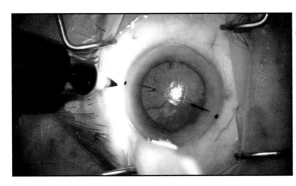

Figure 32-3. After marking the steep postoperative corneal meridian, longer lasting limbal reference marks are placed. Their locations can be adjusted if there was any problem centering the toric marks on the cornea.

Future Methods

It is possible to perform toric IOL implantation without marking the eye at all. The SensoMotoric Instruments surgery guidance system (SMI) produces keratometry readings that are locked to a photograph that contains vessel and other registration landmarks. Because the keratometry readings are locked to the photograph, it is not so critical that the patient's head be positioned perfectly straight in front of the topographer when the keratometry readings are obtained (Figure 32-4). This technology was recently acquired by Alcon Laboratories and will be marketed as the Varion system.

In the operating room, the digital photograph is registered with the live eye. Using an eye tracker and a heads down digital overlay within the operating microscope, a digital steep meridian mark can be placed over the eye that tracks with eye movements. The two marks on the toric IOL are aligned with the digitally generated corneal steep meridian marker. All of this is done without placing a single ink on the eye (Figure 32-5).

Another technology that is gaining momentum is the WaveTec Vision Optiwave Refractive Analysis (ORA) system. This device is an intraoperative aberrometer that attaches to an operating microscope. It measures the refractive state of the eye in the aphakic or pseudophakic state, including sphere and cylinder, and can be used to adjust the axis of a toric IOL in real time. Its limitations are those of all other methods in that it cannot predict the effect of wound healing on final corneal astigmatism, nor the final IOL position after capsule bag contraction. Nevertheless, it is a promising technology.

Figure 32-4. A commercial system locks the keratometry readings to a photograph of the eye.

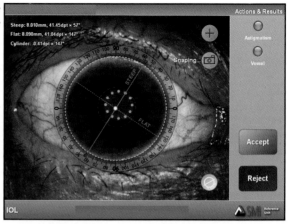

Figure 32-5. Under an operating microscope, the commercial system produces a heads down digital display that tracks with the moving eye and shows the steep postoperative corneal meridian as determined by a toric calculator.

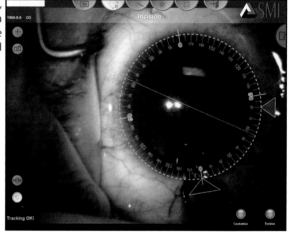

Two new devices just entered the toric alignment market. The first is the Clarity HOLOS IntraOp aberrometer (Pleasanton). It has the potential to provide real-time intraoperative information to guide toric intraocular lens alignment, similar to the WaveTec ORA system. The second is the Callisto eye (Carl Zeiss Meditec). It can create a toric alignment reference in a heads down view within a Zeiss Lumera 700 microscope, similar to the Alcon Verion system. The Callisto eye can operate in two different modes. One requires reference marks to be placed on the limbus at 3 and 9 o'clock (Figure 32-6). The system finds these marks and specifies the corneal meridian for aligning the toric intraocular lens. A markerless system uses the IOLMaster 500 to obtain a reference image and keratometry readings. It then finds the steep postoperative corneal meridian without intraoperative marking, which has obvious surgical efficiency ramifications.

Although not in widespread use at this time, these digital technologies, or something like them, will likely replace current manual techniques that rely on felt tip marking pens.

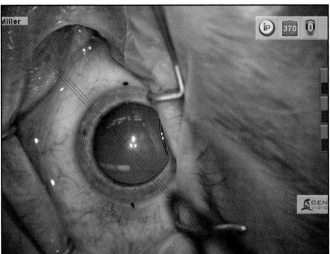

Figure 32-6. Using the original system that requires the placement of limbal reference marks, the Callisto eye identifies the marks place on the horizontal meridian, shown by the yellow line. Next, it identifies the meridian for aligning the toric lens. The system can display a single blue line or three blue lines, as shown here. Three lines are better for dealing with slight displacements of the lens or parallax between the corneal plane and lens plane.

Suggested Readings

Amesbury EC, Miller KM. Approach to the surgical correction of astigmatism at the time of cataract surgery. In: Henderson BA, Gills JP. *A Complete Surgical Guide for Correcting Astigmatism: An Ophthalmic Manifesto*. Thorofare, NJ: SLACK Incorporated; 2010.

Amesbury EC, Miller KM. Correction of astigmatism at the time of cataract surgery. *Curr Opin Ophthalmol*. 2009;20:19-24.

Holland E, Lane S, Horn JD, Ernest P, Arleo R, Miller KM. The AcrySof Toric intraocular lens in subjects with cataracts and corneal astigmatism: A randomized, subject-masked, parallel-group, 1-year study. *Ophthalmology*. 2010;117:2104-2111.

Lane SS, Ernest P, Miller KM, Hileman KS, Harris B, Waycaster CR. Comparison of clinical and patient-reported outcomes with bilateral AcrySof Toric or spherical control intraocular lenses. *J Refract Surg*. 2009;25;899-901.

33
QUESTION

IF A PATIENT HAS RESIDUAL ASTIGMATISM AFTER I IMPLANT A TORIC IOL ON POSTOPERATIVE DAY 1, WHAT SHOULD I DO?

John P. Berdahl, MD

If a patient comes in with residual astigmatism on the day after implantation of a toric intraocular lens (IOL), the first thing you should do is examine the cornea carefully. On the first postoperative day, many factors can lead to residual astigmatism including corneal edema, dryness, wound healing, a slow wound leak, residual pupillary dilation, or a misaligned toric IOL. At this stage, I would not change any treatment course unless the patient has a leaking wound, in which case a suture is warranted. It is very helpful to try to obtain a reliable manifest refraction on the first postoperative day and it is equally important to check the axis of the toric lens that was placed. With the Haag-Streit slit-lamp, the most accurate way to accomplish this is by moving the top portion of the rotating illumination arm of the slit-lamp until the slit-beam is angulated identically to marks on a toric IOL (Figure 33-1). At this point, I would not initiate any treatment, but reassure the patient that I need more time to know the ultimate refraction. I would have the patient return in 1 to 2 weeks to reexamine the eye, repeat a manifest refraction, and recheck the axis of the toric IOL. Next, you should double check to make sure that the axis of placement of the toric IOL is consistent with the axis you intended.

When the patient returns for a 1-week recheck, I would obtain a corneal topography in addition to whichever Ks you used to calculate the toric lens (ie, IOLMaster [Carl Zeiss Inc], Lenstar [Haag-Streit], Manual Ks [Haag-Streit]). Devices like the NIDEK OPD-Scan III or an iTrace (Tracey Technologies LLC) can separate the corneal astigmatism from the intraocular astigmatism (Figure 33-2). However, the two most important measurements to obtain would be a manifest refraction and an accurate measurement of the current axis of the toric IOL. It is critically important that the manifest refraction be accurate. If continued residual astigmatism is present, my next step would be to visit the website www.astigmatismfix.com and input the manifest refraction, which toric IOL was used, and the axis of the toric IOL. The website will calculate if rotating

Henderson BA, Yoo SH. *Curbside Consultation in Refractive and Lens-Based Surgery: 49 Clinical Questions* (pp 129-132)

Figure 33-1. (A) The white dots of varying size that mark off 10-degree increments of rotation. (B) By lining up the angulated slit beam with the marking dots present on the toric IOL, a very accurate estimation of the axis of the toric IOL can be obtained.

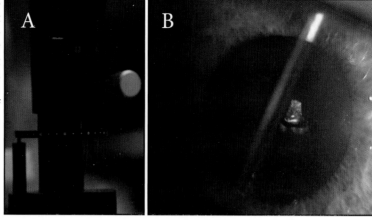

Figure 33-2. A NIDEK OPD-Scan III scan showing the corneal curvature (axial) is neutralized by the internal astigmatism correction of a toric IOL (internal OPD).

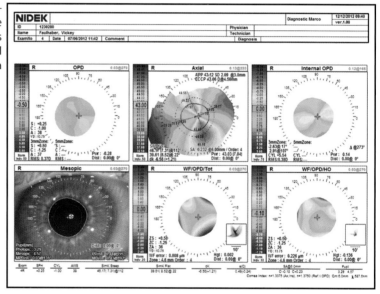

the toric IOL would be beneficial to reduce astigmatism, and how much the toric IOL should be rotated, in addition to the anticipated residual refraction (Figure 33-3). If the cornea appears adequately healed and rotating the IOL would minimize the astigmatism and residual refractive error to an acceptable level, I would bring the patient back to the operating room and rotate the IOL.

The first step is to mark the current axis of the toric IOL with a marking pen on the cornea. Next, I use that as reference point and mark how much the IOL should be rotated from that point (eg, if the IOL rotation is calculated to be 15 degrees clockwise, I mark the IOL axis where it currently is and then place the second marker 15 degrees clockwise from that position) (Figure 33-4). It is important to use the original incisions, if possible, to rotate the IOL. By using the current incisions, no new surgically induced astigmatism should be created. I usually instill intracameral lidocaine, followed by viscoelastic to stabilize the anterior chamber, then open my primary incision. Next, I insert viscoelastic underneath the toric IOL. I carefully advance the viscoelastic cannula along the haptic of the IOL to ensure that the peripheral capsule is widely opened. Then, with a Sinskey hook, I rotate the IOL to the intended position. It is important to remove all viscoelastic from behind the lens. As I am removing the viscoelastic in front of the

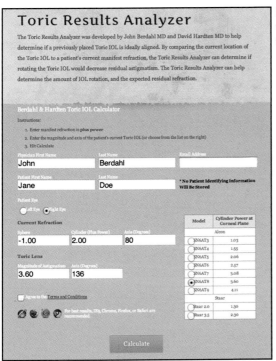

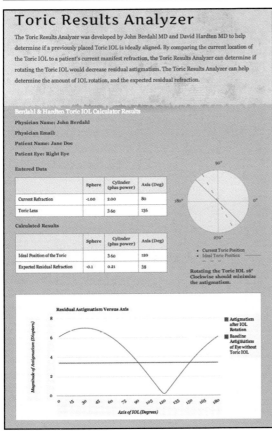

Figure 33-3. Using the Toric Results Analyzer at www.astigmatismfix.com can help determine if the IOL should be rotated.

Figure 33-4. The current position of the toric IOL is marked at the limbus, as is the new position.

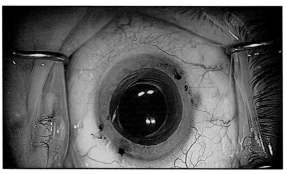

lens, I keep the irrigation and aspiration tip with gentle pressure on the anterior surface of the lens to prevent further rotation. I hydrate the corneal wounds, then I confirm that the IOL is in the intended position. Intraoperative aberrometry can be helpful to confirm the reduction of residual astigmatism as well.

If the patient does not have a spherical equivalent of near plano (or the intended target refraction), then rotating the toric IOL will not result in a satisfactory outcome and the only options are IOL exchange or laser vision correction. In the early postoperative period, I prefer an IOL exchange, but laser vision correction is certainly reasonable.

It is important to understand that the intended axis is not always identical to the ideal axis.

When placing a toric IOL, I almost always rely on anterior corneal curvature; however, I know that posterior corneal curvature plays an important part in the overall refractive state of the eye.[1] Additionally, unanticipated amounts of surgically induced astigmatism will lead to an eye that has residual refractive error.[2] Neither is accounted for in my preoperative plan, but could be accounted for by the use of intraoperative aberrometry.

Ultimately, my goal is hitting a refractive target with little to no residual corneal astigmatism. Ideally, it is nice to rotate the toric lens in the early postoperative period so the anterior and posterior leaflets of the capsular bag have not fused together and around the haptics. It is certainly advisable to rotate the IOL prior to performing a YAG capsulotomy.

As higher powered toric IOLs have become available, and with the future of toric multifocals on the horizon, toric alignment is becoming even more critical.

References

1. Koch DD, Ali SF, Weikert MP, et al. Contribution of posterior corneal astigmatism to total corneal astigmatism. *J Cataract Refract Surg.* 2012;38:2080-2087.
2. Berdahl JP, Hardten DR. Residual astigmatism after toric intraocular lens implantation. *J Cataract Refract Surg.* 2012;38:730.

34
QUESTION

MY ASTIGMATIC KERATOTOMY RESULTS ARE UNPREDICTABLE. HOW CAN I IMPROVE THEM?

R. Bruce Wallace III, MD, FACS

Limbal relaxing incisions (LRIs) are probably the friendliest and most cost-effective refractive procedures we can offer our patients. There is no expensive laser involved, no central corneal or intraocular trauma, and perforations are rare in healthy corneas. So why is it that many cataract surgeons are not yet using LRIs? Some of us are not convinced that they are reliable, especially if, after purchasing the special instruments, the initial results were disappointing. For many, just the awkwardness of incisional corneal surgery along with an uncomfortable change in routine for surgeon and staff have placed LRIs in a negative light. Yet, judging by the swell in attendance at teaching events and LRI wet labs at the last few American Academy of Ophthalmology and American Society of Cataract and Refractive Surgeons meetings, LRIs are growing rapidly in popularity.

We owe a great deal of thanks to early pioneers who promoted the benefits of combining astigmatic keratotomy with cataract surgery many years ago. A partial list would include Drs. Gills, Hollis, Osher, Maloney, Shepherd, Koch, Thornton, Gayton, Davison, and Lindstrom. Dr. Robert Osher has advocated peripheral relaxing keratotomy at the time of cataract surgery since 1983, learning the principles of the technique from Dr. George Tate.[1]

I have had the pleasure of teaching LRI techniques with Drs. Nichamin, Maloney, Dillman, and many others for over 20 years. During these training sessions, I have learned the steps necessary to convince cataract surgeons that LRIs can be an important part of refractive cataract surgery. Before a cataract surgeon transitions to the routine use of LRIs, he or she must do the following:

- Understand the benefits
- Be confident in the "system" of treatment
- Be confident with his or her technique

Henderson BA, Yoo SH. *Curbside Consultation in Refractive and Lens-Based Surgery: 49 Clinical Questions* (pp 133-138)
© 2015 SLACK Incorporated

Treatment Systems

A systematic approach to LRI use improves results. Drs. Gills, Lindstrom, Nichamin, and I have developed a number of LRI nomograms. I first used Dr. Nichamin's excellent nomogram and then modified it to slant more toward one incision for lower levels of cylinder (Tables 34-1 and 34-2). Because we make incisions so far in the corneal periphery, paired incisions were not found to be as important for postoperative corneal regularity as traditional astigmatic keratotomy made at the 6- to 7-mm optical zone (OZ). An advantage of Nichamin nomograms and their modification is that treatment is planned in degrees of arc rather than cord length. Degree measurements are universally more accurate due to the facts that corneal diameters vary and that we make arcs and not straight line incisions.

For lower levels of astigmatism (less than 2.0 D), selecting the axis of cylinder can be challenging.[2] I look at all axis measurements but usually select ones from computerized corneal topography. Sometimes, especially with smaller cylinder corrections, there is poor correlation of the axis as determined by refraction, K readings, and topography. Often when I encounter this situation with first eyes for cataract surgery, I will postpone the LRI and measure the cylinder postoperatively. If there is visually disturbing postoperative astigmatism, I will perform LRIs centered on the axis of the postoperative refraction the same day the patient returns for cataract surgery in the fellow eye. Residual astigmatism in the first eye also alerts me to consider an LRI in the second eye.

Questions arise concerning intraocular lens (IOL) power modifications with LRIs. With low to moderate levels of cylinder (0.50 to 2.75), corneal "coupling" equalizes the central cornea power so there is less chance the IOL power selection will be inaccurate. Longer LRI incisions for higher cylinder (> 3.0 D) may create a radial keratotomy (RK)-like flattening effect and produce unwanted postoperative hyperopia. Increasing the IOL power by 0.5 to 1.0 D may be necessary in these cases.

Instrumentation

Simplification of instruments and techniques improves efficiency and comfort with the procedure. There are many excellent LRI instrument sets available from Mastel, Rhein, Katena, ASICO, and others. I designed the Wallace LRI Kit with Bausch + Lomb–Storz Instruments. This kit includes the following:

- Pre-set single footplate trifacet diamond knife (600 μm)
- Mendez axis marker
- 0.12-caliber forceps

The trifacet diamond is less likely to chip. The Mendez marker has actual numbers on the dial to help guide the surgeon to the proper axis mark. (This orientation guide is valuable because the biggest fear—besides a perforation—is placing the incision in the wrong axis.) All of these instruments are made of titanium to increase longevity.

When using the nomogram, if age/astigmatism at dividing point:

- Choose the shortest incision length
- Choose 1 incision over 2 incisions

Patient Counseling

Similar to preoperative discussion of the new refractive IOLs, informing patients about the option of surgical treatment for astigmatism has become commonplace in many cataract

Table 34-1

Nichamin Age- and Pachymetry-Adjusted (NAPA) Intralimbal Arcuate Astigmatic Nomogram

Preoperative Cylinder, D	Paired Incisions in Degrees of Arc			
	20 to 30 years old	31 to 40 years old	41 to 50 years old	51 to 60 years old
With-the-Rule (Steep Axis 45 to 145 degrees)				
0.75	40	35	35	30
1.00	45	40	40	35
1.25	55	50	45	40
1.50	60	55	50	45
1.75	65	60	55	50
2.00	70	65	60	55
2.25	75	70	65	60
2.50	80	75	70	65
2.75	85	80	75	70
3.00	90	90	85	80
Against-the-Rule (Steep Axis 0 to 40 degrees/140 to 180 degrees)				
0.75	45	40	40	35
1.00	50	45	45	40
1.25	55	55	50	45
1.50	60	60	55	50
1.75	65	65	60	55
2.00	70	70	65	60
2.25	75	75	70	65
2.50	80	80	75	70
2.75	85	85	80	75
3.00	90	90	85	80

When placing intralimbal relaxing incisions following or concomitant with radial relaxing incisions, total arc length is decreased by 50%.
Created by and used with permission from Louis D. "Skip" Nichamin, MD of Laurel Eye Clinic, Brookville, PA.

practices. We start by describing the optical disadvantages of astigmatism and the relative effectiveness and low risk surrounding LRIs. In the United States, when charging Medicare patients

Table 34-2

Limbal Relaxing Incisions: Wallace Nomogram

Instruments

- Diamond knife: Trifacet 600-μm preset depth, single foot plate
- Marker: Mendez axis ring
- Forceps: 0.12 caliber

Procedure

- Place axis ring around limbus.
- Mark axis with forceps.
- Mark limits of intended incision(s) with forceps.
- Remove axis ring.
- Dry marks with cellulose sponge.
- Fixate globe with forceps.
- Perform incision(s), direct toward fixation.

Nomogram

Assuming all cataract incisions are performed temporally and are relatively astigmatically neutral:

Astigmatism, D	40 to 50 years old	50 to 60 years old	60 to 70 years old	70 to 80 years old	80+ years old
For With-the-Rule and Oblique Astigmatism					
1.00 to 1.50	60 degrees[1]	50 degrees[1]	50 degrees[1]	40 degrees[1]	30 degrees[1]
1.50 to 2.00	70 degrees[1]	70 degrees[1]	70 degrees[1]	60 degrees[1]	60 degrees[1]
2.00 to 2.50	60 degrees[2]	60 degrees[2]	60 degrees[2]	70 degrees[1]	70 degrees[1]
2.50 to 3.00	70 degrees[2]	70 degrees[2]	70 degrees[2]	60 degrees[2]	60 degrees[2]
3.00 to 4.00	80 degrees[2]	80 degrees[2]	80 degrees[2]	70 degrees[2]	70 degrees[2]
For Against-the-Rule Astigmatism					
1.00 to 1.50	60 degrees[1]	50 degrees[1]	40 degrees[1]	40 degrees[1]	30 degrees[1]
1.50 to 2.00	70 degrees[1]	60 degrees[1]	60 degrees[1]	60 degrees[1]	40 degrees[1]
2.00 to 2.50	60 degrees[2]	80 degrees[1]	80 degrees[1]	70 degrees[1]	60 degrees[1]
2.50 to 3.00	70 degrees[2]	70 degrees[2]	70 degrees[2]	60 degrees[2]	60 degrees[2]
3.00 to 4.00	80 degrees[2]	80 degrees[2]	80 degrees[2]	70 degrees[2]	70 degrees[2]

[1] denotes 1 incision.
[2] denotes 2 incisions.

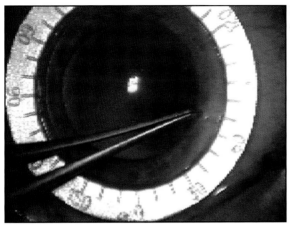

Figure 34-1. Marking the astigmatic axis with a Mendez ring.

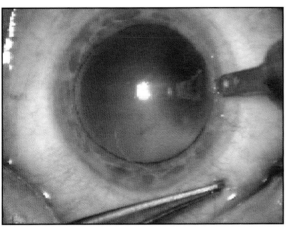

Figure 34-2. LRI placed 1.0 to 1.5 mm from the surgical limbus.

for an additional out-of-pocket fee for LRIs, an advanced beneficiary notice (ABN) should be filed.

Technique

A surgeon's LRI technique will vary depending on the instruments used for the procedure. The routine I use with the Duckworth & Kent instruments is as follows:

1. Make the LRIs before making the phaco incision, but after wetting the cornea.
2. Mark the axis (Mendez ring and 0.12 forceps).
3. Mark the incision borders (Mendez ring and 0.12 forceps).
4. Fixate the globe (0.12 forceps).
5. Advance the knife toward fixation (usually toward the surgeon).

Try to insert the knife into the peripheral corneal dome (approximately 1.5 mm from the actual limbus) as perpendicular as possible (Figures 34-1 and 34-2). Maintain this blade orientation and with moderate pressure complete the LRI by "connecting the dots" on the cornea and twirling the knife handle to make an arcuate incision using the limbus as a template.

Postoperative Care

For many years, I added a nonsteroidal anti-inflammatory drug (NSAID) to our postoperative cataract surgery regimen to offer corneal analgesia. I now use an NSAID routinely for all cataract surgery patients, preoperatively and postoperatively, mainly to help reduce inflammation and the incidence of cystoid macular edema. A topical fourth-generation fluoroquinolone and steroid are also part of my medication routine for cataract surgery. I do not patch the eye after LRIs but do apply povidone-iodine 5% on the cornea preoperatively and immediately postoperatively.

Measuring Results

A number of methods are available to measure results with LRIs. Newer computer software includes postoperative astigmatic analysis. Surgically induced refractive change and vector analysis are often used to demonstrate astigmatic change. A simpler way to follow results is just to measure the amount of postoperative cylinder at any axis. If a patient has <0.75 D of postoperative astigmatism, he or she is likely to be happy with the results.

The Future of Limbal Relaxing Incisions

Like phacoemulsification, LRI instruments and techniques will continue to evolve. As we follow LRI results with imaging such as sophisticated corneal topography and wavefront aberrometry, modifications such as adjustments in blade depth and optic zone diameter will help us improve. Competition with toric IOLs and combinations of bioptics with corneal laser and light adjustable IOLs may reduce LRI popularity. Femtosecond cataract surgery has tended to validate the benefits of LRIs and time will tell as to surgeon adoption of this new technology. In the meantime, traditional LRI techniques remain an important ingredient to achieve spectacle reduction with refractive lens procedures. Regardless, any improvement in methods to reduce unwanted astigmatism will continue to be an important part of successful refractive cataract surgery.

References

1. Osher RH. Consultations in refractive surgery. *J Refract Surg.* 1987;3(6):240.
2. Wallace RB. On-axis cataract incisions: where is the axis? 1995 ASCRS Symposium of Cataract, IOL and Refractive Surgery Best Papers of Sessions. 1995;67-72.

SECTION VI

PRESBYOPIA CORRECTION

35

DO YOU IMPLANT MULTIFOCAL IOLS IN A PATIENT WITH MILD MACULAR DISEASE SUCH AS MILD NON-PROLIFERATIVE DIABETIC RETINOPATHY OR A FEW DRUSEN?

Uday Devgan, MD, FACS, FRCS(Glasg)

Multifocal intraocular lenses (IOLs) provide a wide range of good vision without spectacles by producing two, or sometimes more, focal points within the same optical system. While this doesn't restore youthful accommodation, it does provide a good treatment for presbyopia at the time of cataract surgery. With most multifocal IOLs, this is accomplished by way of diffractive optics to divide the light entering the eye, producing two focal points (Figure 35-1). But this comes at the expense of image quality and contrast sensitivity.

To maximize the visual benefits of a multifocal lens, the eye should have close to a plano post-operative refraction with minimal residual astigmatism. In addition, the other focusing structures should be healthy and normal, such as the cornea and the tear film. Finally, the retina, and in particular the macula, should have normal function and anatomy. Any deficiency in these factors will result in suboptimal vision with a multifocal IOL.

Although patients with mild macular disease, such as mild nonproliferative diabetic retinopathy, can do very well initially with a multifocal IOL, the key issue is the future macular function. Diseases like diabetes are chronic and progressive and we can expect that many patients will slowly develop worsening organ damage over the course of years. The diabetic patient who initially sees quite well with a multifocal IOL may end up with substantial retinal pathology such as clinically significant macular edema (CSME) (Figure 35-2).

Should these patients develop significant retinal disease requiring surgery, the presence of a multifocal IOL may interfere with the intraoperative view for the surgeon. Because these macular changes limit the vision, we want to do everything possible to maximize the optics of the eye, and that means using a monofocal IOL. With any significant macular disease, it is more important to maximize the optics of the eye than it is to provide freedom from spectacles.

Henderson BA, Yoo SH. *Curbside Consultation in Refractive and Lens-Based Surgery: 49 Clinical Questions* (pp 141-143)
© 2015 SLACK Incorporated

Figure 35-1. This patient has a nicely positioned diffractive multifocal lens implanted in the capsular bag after cataract surgery. His visual results were initially excellent, achieving 20/20 distance vision and J1 near vision without the use of spectacles.

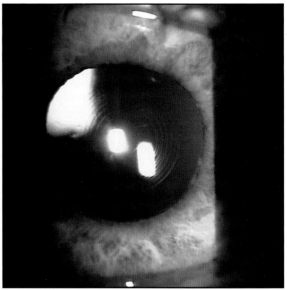

Figure 35-2. The patient had a history of mild nonproliferative diabetic retinopathy without significant macular disease, as seen in this fundus photo. However, over the course of the next few years, he developed worsening retinopathy, including clinically significant macular edema. Despite aggressive laser treatment and intravitreal injections of therapeutic medications, his vision declined and the multifocal IOL further impaired his visual quality, contrast sensitivity, and ability to function.

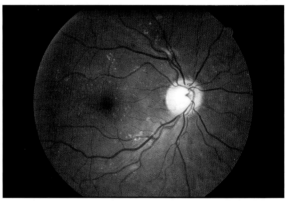

Similarly, patients with mild macular drusen may develop significant age-related macular degeneration (ARMD) in the future. Again, this would limit the benefit of the multifocal IOL and may limit the visual functioning of the patient. Because ARMD is age-related and progressive, we can expect that the incidence of this disease will be higher in older patients and that patients with mild changes have a risk of developing moderate or even severe changes in the future.

Development of cataracts is essentially a certainty in all patients who live long enough, and addressing that with phacoemulsification and IOL implantation is necessary and expected. However, care must be taken to differentiate cataract surgery from refractive surgery, particularly when the latter is accomplished with multifocal IOLs that function best in an otherwise perfectly healthy eye. Because refractive surgery provides visual results that can be achieved with spectacles, it is an elective, even cosmetic procedure that is not required.

The flip side of the argument is that the patient may enjoy many years of excellent vision with the multifocal IOL before developing more significant macular disease. Also, the multifocal IOL could be explanted and exchanged in the future if needed, though performing additional intraocular surgery on an eye with macular edema can result in worsening of the retinal fluid and thickening. Some surgeons have even advocated implanting a multifocal IOL with a −2 diopter (D) myopic postoperative target in patients with ARMD to provide a stronger near addition.

For an eye that is completely healthy and normal, with no signs of chronic conditions that may worsen in the future, a multifocal IOL can be an excellent choice. However, in eyes with early signs of potentially damaging macular disease, a high-quality monofocal IOL may be a better long-term choice. We should keep in mind one of the first lessons we learned in medical school: "First, do no harm."

Bibliography

Gayton JL, Mackool RJ, Ernest PH, Seabolt RA, Dumont S. Implantation of multifocal intraocular lenses using a magnification strategy in cataractous eyes with age-related macular degeneration. *J Cataract Refract Surg.* 2012;38(3):415-418.

Kamath GG, Prasad S, Danson A, Phillips RP. Visual outcome with the array multifocal intraocular lens in patients with concurrent eye disease. *J Cataract Refract Surg.* 2000;26(4):576-581.

Werner L, Olson RJ, Mamalis N. New technology IOL optics. *Ophthalmol Clin North Am.* 2006; 19(4):469-483.

Yoshino M, Inoue M, Kitamura N, Bissen-Miyahima H. Diffractive multifocal intraocular lens interferes with intraoperative view. *Clin Ophthalmol.* 2010;4:467-469.

DO YOU IMPLANT A MULTIFOCAL IOL IN PATIENTS WITH PXF OR OTHER ZONULAR ABNORMALITIES?

Kim-Binh Mai, MD and Bonnie An Henderson, MD

While multifocal intraocular lenses (IOLs) offer a solution to age-related presbyopia, a patient's final visual outcome often depends on a number of factors, including pupillary size,[1-3] corneal astigmatism,[4-6] corneal clarity,[7] and the amount of IOL decentration.[3] Because the natural history of pseudoexfoliation syndrome (PXF) is progressive zonular instability and decreasing pupil size, multifocal IOLs may not achieve their full optical performance in these eyes. Multifocal IOLs are particularly dependent on precise centering[3,8-10] and sufficient pupil size.[1-3] Furthermore, these patients are at risk for poor potential visual outcome secondary to other complications of PXF, such as anterior segment ischemia, glaucoma, and corneal endothelium dysfunction. In some cases, the entire capsular bag/IOL complex may dislocate postoperatively due to zonular dehiscence (Figure 36-1). In a single-center, retrospective study published by Davis et al, PXF was seen in 50% of cases that had spontaneous monofocal IOL dislocation.[11]

In patients with zonular instability but no evidence of PXF, the decision to implant a multifocal IOL should include an assessment of the amount and cause of zonular abnormality. If there is a localized, small area of zonular weakness (approximately less than 3 clock hours), and the cause of zonular weakness is not a progressive or congenital disorder, we will consider implanting a capsular tension ring (CTR), then a multifocal IOL. The CTR will distribute the forces around the equator and help center the multifocal IOL. If a multifocal IOL is implanted, it is important to have a preoperative discussion about the possibility of long-term decentration and possible subluxation.

If a multifocal IOL is significantly displaced from its pupillary center, its optical performance can be adversely affected and lead to decreased uncorrected vision and dysphotopsias.[3] Negishi et al demonstrated that contrast sensitivity was reduced when a multifocal IOL was decentered by 1.0 mm, although visual function was preserved.[8] Several other published experimental studies

Henderson BA, Yoo SH. *Curbside Consultation in Refractive and Lens-Based Surgery: 49 Clinical Questions* (pp 145-147) © 2015 SLACK Incorporated

Figure 36-1. Inferior subluxation of PCIOL and capsular bag complex.

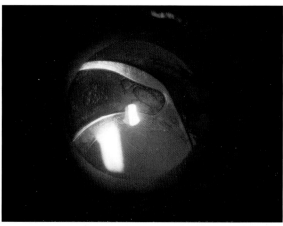

utilizing optical simulation with eye models also replicated similar results regarding the influence of decentration on multifocal IOLs.[9] Soda et al reported that a 1.0-mm decentration of an apodized, diffractive multifocal IOL resulted in an inability to distinguish newspaper characters.[9] This is because when a decentration occurs, a greater proportion of the monofocal area of the periphery is used, while a smaller portion of the diffractive zone near the center (the prime area for near vision) is employed. More recently, Montés-Micó et al measured wavefront aberrations of the studied IOL models and confirmed that decentration and tilting of different aspheric multifocal IOLs did indeed have a significant impact on the optical quality provided by all the multifocal IOLs.[10]

Additional clinical studies analyzing the influence of different degrees of tilt and decentration on the visual performance of patients with multifocal IOLs are needed. Previously published experimental studies are limited because they could not address binocular vision adaptation, nor could they alter the pupil size dynamically.[9] Decentration of 0.3 mm has been observed in uncomplicated monofocal IOL implants,[10] but the amount of decentration in patients with PXF may be significantly higher.

Conclusion

Although PXF and zonular abnormalities are not absolute contraindications, we generally do not recommend a multifocal IOL in these situations because of the unpredictability. However, if a patient has no evidence of phacodonesis preoperatively and is fully aware of the possible risks associated with implanting a multifocal IOL in situations of zonular compromise, then it is reasonable to choose these types of presbyopia-correcting IOLs.

References

1. Hayashi K, Hayashi H, Nakao F, et al. Correlation between pupillary size and intraocular lens decentration and visual acuity of a zonal progressive multifocal lens and a monofocal lens. *Ophthalmology.* 2001;108:2011-2017.
2. Koch DD, Samuelson SW, Haft EA, et al. Pupillary size and responsiveness: Implications for selection of a bifocal intraocular lens. *Ophthalmology.* 1991;98:1030-1035.
3. Koch DD, Samuelson SW, Villarreal R, et al. Changes in pupil size induced by phacoemulsification and posterior chamber lens implantation: Consequences for multifocal lenses. *J Cataract Refract Surg.* 1996;22:579-584.

4. Hayashi K, Hayashi H, Nakao F, et al. Influence of astigmatism on multifocal and monofocal intraocular lenses. *Am J Ophthalmol*. 2000;130:477-482.

5. Jacobi PC, Konen W. Effect of age and astigmatism on the AMO Array multifocal intraocular lens. *J Cataract Refract Surg*. 1995;21:556-561.

6. Ravalico G, Parentin F, Baccara F, et al. Effect of astigmatism on multifocal intraocular lenses. *J Cataract Refract Surg*. 1999;25:804-807.

7. Dick HB, Krummenauer F, Schwenn O, et al. Objective and subjective evaluation of photic phenomena after monofocal and multifocal intraocular lens implantation. *Ophthalmology*. 1999;106:1878-1886.

8. Negishi K, Ohnuma K, Ikeda T, Noda T. Visual simulation of retina images through a decentered monofocal and a refractive multifocal intraocular lens. *J Jpn Ophthalmol Soc*. 2005;49:281-286.

9. Soda M, Yaguchi S. Effect of decentration on the optical performance in multifocal intraocular lenses. *Ophthalmologica*. 2012;227:197-204.

10. Montés-Micó R, López-Gil N, Pérez-Vives C, et al. In vitro optical performance of nonrotational symmetric and refractive–diffractive aspheric multifocal intraocular lenses: Impact of tilt and decentration. *J Cataract Refract Surg*. 2012;38:1657-1663.

11. Davis D, Brubaker J, Espandar L, et al. Late-in-the-bag spontaneous intraocular lens dislocation: Evaluation of 86 consecutive cases. *Ophthalmology*. 2009;116(4):664-670.

37

DESCRIBE YOUR APPROACH IN COUNSELING A PATIENT REGARDING THE "PREMIUM" IOL CHOICES. DO YOU DELEGATE THE RESPONSIBILITY?

Richard L. Lindstrom, MD; Sumitra S. Khandelwal, MD;
David R. Hardten, MD; and Sherman Reeves, MD

In our practice, the surgeon takes the primary responsibility to discuss intraocular lens (IOL) options with the patient at the cataract evaluation, but our entire team is educated about the features and potential benefits of premium IOL implantation.

Prior to examination, patients are asked to fill out a form that asks about their preferred refractive targets. We find this is helpful, as often patients have not thought about this aspect of their surgery.

Our practice has used several different forms in the past, but we have found that simpler is better. Currently, we ask patients to choose which they prefer from the following 4 options:

1. Mostly distance

2. Mostly near

3. Both far and near

4. I don't mind wearing glasses for all distances

In addition, if it is known that the patient has a cataract, a brochure explaining the diagnosis of cataract and lens implant options is mailed to the patient. We also have a considerable amount of educational material on our website, including surgeon discussion, videos, and the animations from eye examinations.

Following the clinical examination, if cataract surgery in indicated, the surgeon will complete an informed consent discussion, including the choices for IOL. We like to describe the possibility of a lifestyle-enhancing reduction in spectacle dependence as an opportunity we want the patient to consider. We do not try to sell the patient on any specific IOL and are careful to make sure we leave the impression that a monofocal IOL is an excellent option.

Henderson BA, Yoo SH. *Curbside Consultation in Refractive and Lens-Based Surgery: 49 Clinical Questions* (pp 149-151)
© 2015 SLACK Incorporated

We discuss monofocal lenses and the advantages of high-quality vision and reduced cost. We make it clear that it provides a single focus, does not correct astigmatism, and is limited to one focal point. Following that, discussion of premium lenses will begin. If the patient has astigmatism, we discuss toric lenses, corneal relaxing incisions, and laser surgery following cataract surgery.

For presbyopia correction lenses, our practice uses mostly Tecnis Multifocal Lens (Abbott Medical Optics Inc), but we also do monovision and have Crystalens (Bausch + Lomb) and ReSTOR (Alcon Inc) available for select patients if they do not want to wear reading glasses.

The surgeon will describe the advantage of achieving functional near and distance vision with reduced dependence on glasses. In addition, he or she will discuss the possible glare and halos, and intermediate focal point limitations. We also discuss the possibility that there is a "neuroadaptation" to one's new vision after surgery, and that a small number of patients do not adapt well and could require an IOL exchange.

Lastly, we discuss that premium lenses require precise refractive outcomes to function at their maximum, and additional testing, intraoperative techniques, and even postoperative laser enhancements may be necessary. We offer refractive enhancements with excimer laser following premium lenses.

We believe it is important at this time to let patients have time to think about the options. We have them meet with a surgical coordinator, who will review the options again, and discuss tier options and pricing. If the patient wishes to think about it and discuss with family, we offer the opportunity to call back with any questions for the surgeon in regards to lens choice or to the surgical counselors in regards to cost.

Once the patient decides on his or her preference, the final decision is recorded in the chart so that on the day of surgery there is no confusion as to what tier and type of lens the patient has selected. The surgeon then confirms this decision just prior to surgery with the patient and family. Fees are collected prior to surgery.

Non-Candidates

We try to discuss lens options with every patient we evaluate, even if he or she does not qualify for a premium IOL. For these patients, the surgeon explains, "There are many different lens options including some lenses that can focus distance and near; however, because of your (insert pathology), this would not be a good lens choice for you." We do this so that patients do not hear about the lenses from a friend or on the Internet and wonder why we did not offer it for them. Once patients hear that they are not candidates for a premium IOL, they can open their minds to monofocal lenses.

Comanagement

Because we comanage a number of patients in regards to cataract surgery with referring ophthalmologists and optometrists, some of whom come from quite a distance, there are times where the referring provider has discussed lens options. For those referring providers with whom we work closely, it is preferred that they initiate the discussion with the patient and address the patient's request in the referring letter.

That being said, our surgeons still have the discussion with the patient again, especially if he or she wishes to have a premium lens. In particular, there are times when a patient requests a multifocal IOL, but there is something about his or her exam that precludes the patient from that lens. It is a delicate discussion, but as much time as needed is taken to assure that the patient and referring doctor are comfortable and understand the final decision on lens implant.

Conclusion

Patient satisfaction is very high with premium lenses, but part of the process must be excellent communication and service. We believe having the surgeon personally discuss the options is important.

A successful premium lens practice requires a "high touch/high tech" approach. Additional time is required of the surgeon and staff, and additional technology is needed to generate the outcomes required for high patient satisfaction. All of our technicians, nurses, optometrists, medical ophthalmologists, and surgical counselors are fully educated about the lens alternatives. We believe the outcomes justify the effort, and highly satisfied patients and referring doctors are key drivers of our practice's success.

Suggested Readings

Barsam A, Voldman A, Donnenfeld E. Advanced technology IOLs in cataract surgery: Management of the unhappy patient. *Int Ophthalmol Clin*. 2012;52(2):95-102.

Davis EA, Hardten DR, Lindstrom RL. *Presbyopic Lens Surgery: A Clinical Guide to Current Technology*. Thorofare NJ: SLACK Incorporated; 2007.

Lichtinger A, Rootman DS. Intraocular lenses for presbyopia correction: Past, present, and future. *Curr Opin Ophthalmol*. 2012;23(1):40-46.

QUESTION

38

WHAT ARE THE INDICATIONS FOR MONOVISION VS OTHER PRESBYOPIA-CORRECTING IOL OPTIONS? HOW MUCH ANISOMETROPIA IS ADVISABLE WITH MONOVISION WITH MONOFOCAL IOLS?

Wei Boon Khor, MBBS, FRCSEd and Natalie Afshari, MD, FACS

Monovision is an optical technique to correct presbyopia; typically, the dominant eye is corrected for distance vision, while the fellow eye is optimized for near vision.[1] This technique has been used successfully with contact lenses,[1] corneal refractive surgery,[2] and with monofocal intraocular lenses (IOLs) during cataract surgery (pseudophakic monovision).[3]

When we discuss cataract surgery with patients, we routinely ask about their expectations for near vision after the surgery. Many patients are motivated to reduce their dependence on spectacles after cataract surgery, and it is important to provide them with the available options. In our practice, this would include the use of multifocal or accommodative IOLs or pseudophakic monovision with monofocal IOLs. As with any form of refractive surgery, careful patient selection is necessary to achieve a good outcome. We would consider the following patients to be better candidates for pseudophakic monovision over presbyopia-correcting IOLs:

- Patients with prior experience with monovision (through contact lens wear or as a result of refractive surgery) who were happy with the results

- Patients who are accepting of some decreased stereopsis and contrast sensitivity with monovision, and are not adverse to wearing spectacles for specific activities (eg, night driving)

- Patients with cost considerations, as presbyopia-correcting IOLs usually require additional out-of-pocket expenses

There are other groups of patients with whom we would also discuss the use of monovision:

- *Postcorneal refractive surgery*: In patients with previous corneal refractive surgery, especially those with dysphotic phenomena such as halos and glare, we would avoid the use of multifocal IOLs because of the risk of exacerbating such symptoms. Although accommodative IOLs are a

Henderson BA, Yoo SH. *Curbside Consultation in Refractive and Lens-Based Surgery: 49 Clinical Questions* (pp 153-155)
© 2015 SLACK Incorporated

possibility, we have not found them to perform well in our hands. For these patients, we would carefully discuss the use of monovision in order to reduce spectacle dependence.

- *Occupational needs*: For patients who work or perform at night or in low-light conditions (eg, radiologists, cab drivers), we would generally avoid the use of multifocal IOLs given the possible dysphotic side effects and reduced contrast sensitivity. Although monovision is an option, we do emphasize that patients may need to wear spectacles to fully correct their binocular vision during work because monovision can also give rise to decreased contrast sensitivity and visual acuity under these lighting conditions. Some patients can and do accept this compromise in order to be spectacle independent outside of work.

While pseudophakic monovision is generally quite suitable for most patients, we would caution against this technique in the following patients (and this is not an exhaustive list):

- Patients who were previously *not* able to adapt to monovision

- Patients with a history of amblyopia, which implies strong sighting preference on one eye over another

- Patients with large phorias, especially if there are symptoms of asthenopia or intermittent diplopia, because the phoria may decompensate after surgery due to the disruption in binocular fusion

- Patients with unrealistic expectations of complete spectacle independence after surgery

With monovision, our refractive target for the patient would be emmetropia for the dominant eye, and typically –2.00 diopters (D) for the nondominant eye. We find that –2.00 D allows most of our patients to read a book or newspaper comfortably, although prolonged reading of fine print may still require a pair of readers. Furthermore, anisometropia of –2.00 D is generally tolerable to most patients after a period of adaptation. However, with the widespread use of computers at work and at home, some patients who rely mainly on "computer vision" may benefit from a myopic correction of –1.00 D in the nondominant eye.

In order to achieve these target refractions, the preoperative assessment should include precise keratometry and biometry, and the use of appropriate lens power formulas with optimized IOL constants; this is particularly important for patients who have undergone corneal refractive surgery. Eyes with astigmatism greater than –1.0 D should be corrected as well as possible (eg, with limbal relaxing incisions, toric IOLs) so that the quality of monovision is not reduced.

The cataract surgery should be performed meticulously to avoid any intraoperative complications; in particular, a capsular rupture may require the placement of the IOL in the sulcus or in the anterior chamber, and give rise to further variability in the postoperative refractive outcome.

We occasionally encounter a patient who is dissatisfied with the results of pseudophakic monovision after surgery, due to a refractive surprise in one or both eyes after surgery. Other patients find that they cannot adapt to monovision despite achieving the refractive targets, and this may be due to difficulties with interocular suppression of the two disparate images, or conversely, due to a strong sighting preference in one eye over the other. Patients must be counseled preoperatively regarding such possibilities, but we am also prepared to intervene if they do arise. Some patients can accept the use of spectacles to correct the refractive error or anisometropia; for others, surgical options such as corneal refractive surgery (our preference would be photorefractive keratectomy), or rarely, an IOL exchange, may be necessary to optimize or reverse the monovision effect.

References

1. Jain S, Arora I, Azar DT. Success of monovision in presbyopes: Review of the literature and potential applications to refractive surgery. *Surv Ophthalmol.* 1996;40(6):491-499.

2. Torricelli AA, Junior JB, Santhiago MR, Bechara SJ. Surgical management of presbyopia. *Clin Ophthalmol.* 2012;6:1459-1466.

3. Ito M, Shimizu K, Iida Y, Amano R. Five-year clinical study of patients with pseudophakic monovision. *J Cataract Refract Surg.* 2012;38(8):1440-1445.

How Do You Choose Between a Multifocal and an Accommodating IOL?

Jay S. Pepose, MD, PhD

There are three essential steps that help guide the ophthalmologist in advising patients who are deciding between accommodating and multifocal intraocular lens (IOL) options. This premium group of lens implants has sometimes been referred to as "lifestyle IOLs." Appropriately, the first step in the decision tree is taking the time to understand each individual's lifestyle, functional needs, and expectations. Each presbyopia-correcting IOL has inherent strengths and weaknesses. IOL design features that achieve an expanded through-focus often are counterbalanced by some limitations or unwanted side effects. Understanding the inherent optical performance of each specific accommodating or multifocal IOL and balancing this with the patient's lifestyle and visual priorities is the second critical step in this iterative process.

The final step in the determination is appreciating each individual's distinctive ocular traits and characteristics, which may impact the performance of an IOL in that individual. Examples of this step include evaluating pupil size, shape and dynamics, corneal wavefront, angle kappa, and macular status.

Step 1: Understanding the Patient's Lifestyle and Shaping His or Her Expectations

Every refractive lens surgeon understands that there is no pseudophakos that mimics the elegant fusion of form and function of an 18-year-old's crystalline lens. Although with time we have seen iterative improvements in accommodating and multifocal IOL design, empathizing with patients that unfortunately there is no "perfect" man-made substitute for the lens they were

Henderson BA, Yoo SH. *Curbside Consultation in Refractive and Lens-Based Surgery: 49 Clinical Questions* (pp 157-161) © 2015 SLACK Incorporated

given by their creator aligns you with patients as their honest advisor and advocate. Starting out by sharing this simple but important acknowledgment of the limitations of current IOL technology in comparison to the youthful crystalline lens goes a long way toward setting the stage for realistic expectations, the need for some compromise with either a multifocal or accommodating IOL, along with our inability to promise or guarantee total spectacle independence at all object vergences and lighting conditions. Within this framework, a very important part of the decision between a specific multifocal vs accommodating IOL is dependent on the patient's lifestyle, visual needs, and expectations, which can best be assessed with a series of open-ended questions.

Patients should be required to rank in order and priority their desire for optimized uncorrected distance, intermediate, and near vision. While everyone would naturally want "perfect" vision at all vergences and almost everyone would be dissatisfied without good uncorrected distance vision, patients should be asked if they frequently use a computer or smartphone or perform other intermediate tasks. With regard to near vision, do the patients enjoy knitting or fly fishing or have other particularly close visual needs? How close does he or she hold things when reading? Would patients consider the need for reading glasses for smaller print a failure of IOL implantation? Do patients frequently drive after dark? Note that the way this question is posed is important, in that patients may initially state that they do little "night driving" until reminded that it is dark as early as 5 pm in the fall. Would some degree of halos around point sources of light at night be an acceptable or completely unacceptable exchange for improved uncorrected near vision? Is the patient currently emmetropic, hyperopic, or myopic, and how does this impact his or her postoperative expectations of uncorrected vision at various distances? In the next section, we see how the answers to these questions bring the doctor to the second step in optimizing the selection of the multifocal or accommodating IOL to best meet each patient's needs.

Step 2: Matching the Patient's Visual Needs to Intraocular Lens Performance, Limitations, and Side Effects

Clinical and optical bench studies both demonstrate important differences in the performance of accommodating vs specific multifocal IOL at various vergences.[1,2] A prospective study of patients randomized to bilateral implantation of the Crystalens AO (Bausch + Lomb) vs ReSTOR 3.0 (Alcon Laboratories) vs Tecnis multifocal IOL (Abbott Medical Optics) demonstrated that patients implanted with Crystalens achieved a better uncorrected and best corrected intermediate vision at 32 inches compared with either multifocal.[3] In contrast to the accommodating IOL, patients implanted with either multifocal achieved better uncorrected and best corrected near vision. The near focal point of the Tecnis multifocal (~31 to 33 cm)[4,5] is closer than the ReSTOR 3.0 (~37 cm)[6] because the Tecnis has a 4.0-diopter (D) add compared with the ReSTOR's 3.0 D add at the IOL plane. However, because the diffractive elements on the Tecnis are on the posterior surface of the IOL in contrast to the ReSTOR apodized rings on the anterior surface, this serves to push the Tecnis' near point farther out than the near point on the ReSTOR 4.0 (~31 cm), yet closer than the ReSTOR 3.0. Objective and subjective tests of glare and halos show that these are greater with the Tecnis than the ReSTOR and least with Crystalens AO.[3]

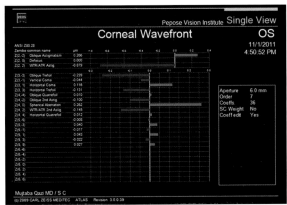

Figure 39-1. Metrics of horizontal and vertical coma, spherical aberration, and other higher-order aberrations are readily quantified in this Zernike decomposition of the corneal wavefront at a 6-mm zone performed using a Zeiss Atlas topographer.

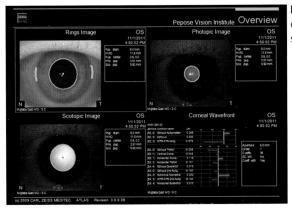

Figure 39-2. The same topography unit also quantifies the pupil diameter and shows its shape under mesopic and photopic conditions.

Step 3: Matching the Patient's Ocular Traits and Characteristics to Specific Intraocular Lens Performance

The performance of both accommodating and multifocal IOLs depends on a number of factors. Residual defocus and astigmatism impacts the function of all IOLs, but comparative clinical and bench studies have shown that both distance and near vision are generally more affected in patients with multifocal IOLs with 0.75 D or more of residual astigmatism.[2] Similarly, image quality in eyes implanted with multifocal IOLs is adversely affected by high degrees of higher-order aberrations, such as coma and spherical aberration. A number of topographers and combined topography/wavefront systems are capable of assessing the corneal wavefront preoperatively. Patients with greater than 0.3 microns of vertical or horizontal coma at a 6-mm optical zone may not be ideal candidates for multifocal IOLs (Figure 39-1) because this may be associated with glare, waxy vision, and reduced image quality.

The performance of apodized diffractive IOLs such as ReSTOR is very dependent on changes in pupil size to shift light energy from near to far foci. It is important to assess pupil size, shape, and dynamics preoperatively (Figure 39-2), in that patients with small, miotic, poorly reactive pupils in both mesopic and photopic conditions may have light energy chronically shifted toward near foci and elicit a waxy distance image quality. Conversely, patients with very large pupils that do not constrict well on accommodation may not achieve the near vision that they are seeking with a ReSTOR multifocal. Although the Tecnis multifocal splits light evenly between near and far at all pupil diameters and may thereby allow reading vision even in lower illumination, studies have shown that intermediate vision is worse in patients with the Tecnis IOL, with pupils ≥ 4 mm compared with those with smaller pupils.[4,5]

Angle kappa[7] is defined clinically as the angular distance in object space between the line of sight (ie, line connecting the pupillary center and the fixation point) and the pupillary axis (ie, the line passing through the center of the pupil perpendicular to the cornea). A prospective study of patients with refractive multifocal IOLs showed that patients' complaints of glare and halos were positively correlated with preoperative values of angle kappa.[8] One explanation for this observation is that if angle kappa is greater than half the diameter of the central optical zone of a multifocal IOL, the primary path of light may traverse one of the multifocal rings instead of the central optic, leading to glare. The ReSTOR 3.0 IOL has a central optical zone of 0.8 mm and the Tecnis MF has a central optical zone of 1 mm. As a reasonable referent value, it may be that an angle kappa of less than 0.4 mm for ReSTOR 3.0 and 0.5 mm for Tecnis MF would greatly lessen the chances of the primary ray traversing the diffractive ring.

Because multifocal IOLs may, in some patients, reduce contrast sensitivity when the light energy is split between near and distance images simultaneously cast on the retina, patients with other independent reasons to have reduced contrast sensitivity may not be ideal candidates for multifocal IOLs. For example, contrast sensitivity may be reduced in patients with current comorbidities such as epiretinal membranes, macular degeneration, myopic degeneration, diabetic retinopathy, dry eye disease, and glaucoma, or in individuals who develop these conditions with age. In comparison, accommodating IOLs have not been shown to reduce contrast sensitivity when compared with aspheric monofocal control IOLs.

Integrating the Results of the Three-Step Process in Surgical Planning

The final recommendation between a specific multifocal or accommodating IOL involves integrating and synthesizing all of the information that has been accumulated. For example, patients who do little night driving and whose main interests are knitting and watching television may be ideally suited for a Tecnis multifocal IOL, if they can accept the possibility of some halos and night glare, which may diminish somewhat with neuroadaptation over the course of months. Patients who work in low lighting conditions, such as a waiter in a low-lit restaurant, an x-ray technologist, or someone who hunts at dusk, may not achieve adequate near vision with a ReSTOR IOL and may not be accepting of photic phenomenon or night glare with a Tecnis or ReSTOR. Such patients might be offered a Crystalens accommodating IOL with some degree of myopic offset of the nondominant eye up to approximately –0.75 D, with the warning that they may still require reading glasses. Patients with 4-mm mesopic pupils that react briskly to accommodation and who spend a lot of time on computers and read frequently may find that the Tecnis IOL gives a closer near point than their computer monitor (requiring them to move the screen closer or use low add readers), and may be better candidates for either a ReSTOR 3.0 or Crystalens with a myopic offset of the nondominant eye to mini-monovision.

Listening to patients' needs, appropriately modifying their expectations, and assessing their ocular traits allows the ophthalmologist to synthesize this information and to use the aforementioned framework as a decision tree in choosing between a multifocal and accommodating IOL.

References

1. Pepose JS, Wang D, Altmann GE. Comparison of through-focus image sharpness across five presbyopia-correcting intraocular lenses. *Am J Ophthalmol.* 2012;154:20-28.
2. Zheleznyak L, Kim MJ, MacRae S, Yoon G. Impact of corneal aberrations on through-focus image quality of presbyopia-correcting intraocular lenses using an adaptive optics bench system. *J Cataract Refract Surg.* 2012; 38:1724-1733.
3. Pepose JS, Qazi MA, Chu R, Stahl J. A prospective randomized clinical evaluation of three presbyopia-correcting intraocular lenses following cataract extraction. *Am J Ophthalmol.* 2014; In press.
4. Hütz WW, Eckhardt HB, Röhrig B, Grolmus R. Intermediate vision and reading speed with Array, Tecnis, and ReSTOR intraocular lenses. *J Refract Surg.* 2008;24:251-256.
5. Packer P, Chu YR, Waltz KL, et al. Evaluation of the aspheric Tecnis multifocal intraocular lens: One-year results from the first cohort of the Food and Drug Administration clinical trial. *Am J Ophthalmol.* 2010;149:577-584.
6. Maxwell WA, Cionni RJ, Lehmann RP, Modi SS. Functional outcomes after bilateral implantation of apodized diffractive aspheric acrylic intraocular lenses with a +3.0 or +4.0 diopter addition power. Randomized multicenter clinical study. *J Cataract Refract Surg.* 2009;35:2054-2061.
7. Park CY, Oh SY, Chuck RS. Measurement of angle kappa and centration in refractive surgery. *Curr Opin Ophthalmol.* 2012;23:269-275.
8. Prakash G, Prakash DR, Agarwal A, Kumar DA, Agarwal A, Jacob S. Predictive factor and kappa angle analysis for visual satisfaction in patients with multifocal IOL implantation. *Eye.* 2011;25:1187-1193.

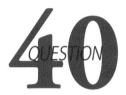

IS A MONOCULAR IMPLANTATION OF A MULTIFOCAL IOL TOLERATED?

Kimiya Shimizu, MD, PhD and Yoshihiko Iida, MD, PhD

Presbyopic cataract surgery encompasses several methods used to compensate for the loss of accommodation by implanting an intraocular lens (IOL). Current approaches include multifocal and accommodating IOLs and the application of the monovision method. The most popular method for presbyopic cataract surgery is bilateral implantation of multifocal IOLs. Recently, various multifocal IOL styles have become available. Many studies have compared distance acuity between multifocal and monofocal IOLs and reported superior near and intermediate vision with multifocal IOLs.

However, multifocal IOLs have several limitations: in particular, visual outcomes with refractive multifocal IOLs vary depending on the pupil diameter. The optical design of refractive or diffractive multifocal IOLs can cause glare and halo symptoms and decrease contrast sensitivity. Some patients with multifocal IOLs report waxy vision (ie, a feeling of looking through water). These problems cannot be solved by eyeglasses or contact lenses because of the limited optical quality of multifocal IOLs.

Monovision (another method of presbyopic correction) with contact lenses was first described by Fonda in 1966.[1] The monovision approach for presbyopic cataract surgery has been used since 1999,[2] and ocular dominance as well as patient satisfaction and visual performance with pseudophakic monovision have been reported. Higher patient satisfaction with pseudophakic monovision is related to excellent uncorrected distance visual acuity (UDVA) in the dominant eye. Monofocal IOLs reportedly have advantages over multifocal IOLs in achieving excellent UDVA and contrast sensitivity.

Taken together, we believe that monocular (particularly, the nondominant eye) implantation is better than binocular implantation.

We report two cases of monocular implantation of multifocal IOLs.

Henderson BA, Yoo SH. *Curbside Consultation in Refractive and Lens-Based Surgery: 49 Clinical Questions* (pp 163-165)
© 2015 SLACK Incorporated

Figure 40-1. Comparison of perioperative pattern visually evoked cortical potentials (P-VECPs) for two patients. P-VECPs were recorded with binocular pattern-reversal stimulation and the results displayed in a double trace. After IOL exchange in the dominant eye, P-VECP amplitude increased and peak latency improved. (Reprinted with permission from Shimizu, K, Ito, M. Dissatisfaction after bilateral multifocal intraocular lens implantation: an electrophysiology study. *Journal of Refractive Surgery.* 2011;27(4).)

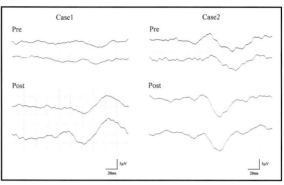

Intraocular Lens Exchange

In cases of unclear vision (eg, waxy vision) resulting from bilateral implantation of multifocal IOLs, a multifocal IOL is exchanged for a monofocal IOL in the dominant eye. The dominant eye is determined by the hole-in-card test. The relationship between dissatisfaction and pattern visually evoked cortical potential (P-VECP) was analyzed.[3]

Intraocular Lens Exchange in the Dominant Eyes of Two Patients

These eyes were implanted with diffractive multifocal IOLs bilaterally. Binocular distant and near visual acuity were 25/20 and 20/20, respectively. They did not show dry eye syndrome, macular edema, posterior capsule opacification, or IOL decentration. Despite good binocular visual acuity for more than 6 months after surgery, these patients showed persistent dissatisfaction with the quality and sharpness of vision even after using spectacles and contact lenses.

To resolve this problem, we exchanged the multifocal IOL in the dominant eye for a monofocal IOL. After surgery, binocular distant and near visual acuities were 30/20 and 20/20, respectively. The amplitude of the P100 component of P-VECP increased and the peak latency improved. The symptoms improved and the patients were satisfied with the visual quality (Figure 40-1).

Thus, in cases that require exchange of multifocal IOL for monofocal IOLs, IOL exchange in the dominant eye is recommended.

Hybrid Monovision

We suggest a presbyopia correcting technique in which a monofocal IOL and multifocal IOL are implanted in the dominant eye and contralateral nondominant eye, respectively, a method we call "hybrid monovision."[4] The exclusion criteria were corneal astigmatism greater than 1.00 D, strabismus, and ocular disease other than cataract.

Figure 40-2 shows the UDVA results in 32 patients at a postoperative follow-up of 3 months. The mean binocular visual acuity at all distances was at least 0.10 logMAR.

The binocular results from intermediate-to-far (0.5 to 5.0 m) vision were significantly better than the monocular results (0.5 m, 0.7 m, and 3.0 m, $P < .01$; 5.0 m, $P < .05$).

Figure 40-3 shows the contrast sensitivity results. In the nondominant eye with the multifocal IOL, contrast sensitivity was decreased at all spatial frequencies. In binocular vision, contrast sensitivity was increased. In the intermediate-to-high spatial frequency ranges (6 to 18 cycles per degree), binocular summation was observed ($P < .01$). No glare, halo, or waxy vision was recorded.

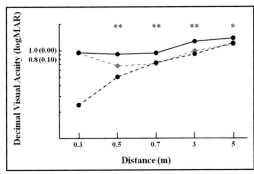

Figure 40-2. Binocular visual acuity is better than 0.10 logMAR at all distances. *P<.05, **P<.01, Wilcoxon signed-rank test; solid black line, binocular; broken black line, dominant eye; broken gray line, nondominant eye. (Reprinted from *Journal of Cataract & Refractive Surgery*, 37(11), Iida Y, Shimizu K, Ito M, Pseudophakic monovision using monofocal and multifocal intraocular lenses: hybrid monovision, Copyright 2011 with permission from Elsevier.)

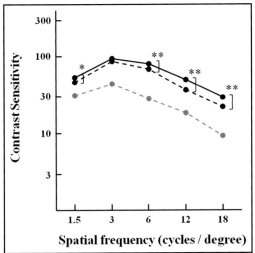

Figure 40-3. Contrast sensitivity. *P<.05, **P<.01, Wilcoxon signed-rank test; solid black line, binocular; broken black line, dominant eye; broken gray line, nondominant eye. (Reprinted from *Journal of Cataract & Refractive Surgery*, 37(11), Iida Y, Shimizu K, Ito M, Pseudophakic monovision using monofocal and multifocal intraocular lenses: hybrid monovision, Copyright 2011 with permission from Elsevier.)

Most surgeons advocate bilateral multifocal IOL implantation to achieve improved visual function. Bilateral implantation should be discussed before surgery. If cataract surgery is performed in one eye alone, the dominant eye is determined by the hole-in-card test; accordingly, a multifocal IOL or a monofocal IOL is selected for the nondominant or dominant eye.

Monocular implantation of multifocal IOLs (in the nondominant eye) is an effective approach for presbyopic cataract surgery using multifocal IOLs. Furthermore, implantation of monofocal IOLs in the dominant eye (hybrid monovision) may reduce glare and halo. In cases of unclear vision, such as waxy vision resulting from bilateral implantation of multifocal IOLs, IOL exchange in the dominant eye is recommended.

References

1. Fonda G. Presbyopia corrected with single vision spectacles or corneal lenses in preference to bifocal corneal lenses. *Trans Am Opthalmol Soc.* 1966;25:78-80.
2. Ito M, Shimizu K, Iida Y, Amano R. Five-year clinical study of patients with pseudophakic monovision. *J Cataract Refract Surg.* 2012;38:1440-1445.
3. Shimizu K, Ito M. Dissatisfaction after bilateral multifocal intraocular lens implantation: an electrophysiology study. *J Refract Surg.* 2011;27:309-312.
4. Iida Y, Shimizu K, Ito M. Pseudophakic monovision using monofocal and multifocal intraocular lenses: Hybrid monovision. *J Cataract Refract Surg.* 2011;37:2001-2005.

IS CHECKING FOR EYE DOMINANCE IMPORTANT? IF SO, WHY, AND WHAT IS YOUR METHOD?

Jae Yong Kim, MD, PhD

Eye dominance is the tendency to prefer visual input from one eye over the other, or functional lateralization.[1] It is very important to check for this type of dominance in clinical and surgical situations. Ophthalmologists should bear in mind the importance of eye dominance when considering both monovision and unilateral refractive correction using lenses and cataract/refractive surgeries. When monovision is created for the presbyopic patient in whom the dominant eye is conventionally corrected for distance vision and the nondominant eye is corrected for near vision,[2] it is critical to know which eye is dominant. Eye dominance should always be assessed prior to any treatment or therapy initiation. If the dominant eye becomes blurred or distorted by cataract or retinal problems, for example, it is common to switch to the nondominant eye. Additionally, several surgical procedures for the healthy presbyopic eyes, such as conductive keratoplasty and corneal inlay insertion, are usually performed only on the nondominant eye.[3,4] When performing refractive surgery or implantation of premium intraocular lens (IOL) in both eyes, it is first completed in the nondominant eye in order to achieve the best refractive outcome in the dominant eye later. However, in case of myopic refractive surgery for monovision, it is first completed in the dominant eye in order to assess the patient's ability to adapt to the monovision condition. The mixing and matching technique, in which two different designs of multifocal IOLs are implanted, can provide patients with the best range of vision without significant visual complications.[5] IOLs demonstrating better near vision are ReSTOR 4+ SN6AD3 (Alcon Laboratories), Tecnis ZM900 (Advanced Medical Optics [AMO], Inc), and Acri.Lisa 366D (Zeiss) IOLs that are equal to or greater than +3.75 near addition, whereas IOLs that display better intermediate vision are ReSTOR +3 SN6AD3, Rezoom (AMO, Inc), and Lentis M plus LS-312 (Oculentis GmbH, Inc).

During preparation for bilateral cataract surgery using the mixing and matching technique, we ask patients for their preferred working distance. It is usually recommended that the IOLs with

Henderson BA, Yoo SH. *Curbside Consultation in Refractive and Lens-Based Surgery: 49 Clinical Questions* (pp 167-169)
© 2015 SLACK Incorporated

Figure 41-1. Checking eye dominance.

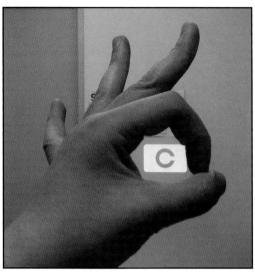

better intermediate vision should be implanted in the dominant eye, and the IOLs with better near vision be implanted in the nondominant eye. If the patient prefers near working distances, both IOLs are reversely implanted.

Eye dominance is checked with the simple "hole-in-the-card" test. Dr. Stahl has described this method in detail in his article regarding conductive keratoplasty.[4] First, the examinee is instructed to sit with shoulders and feet square to a 20/400 Snellen E chart in the examination room and given an 8¾ × 4¾-inch card containing a 1¼-inch hole in the center. Next, keeping both eyes open and observing the 20/400 E target, the patient holds the card horizontally at arm's length and centers the card just below the target. The patient then raises the card so that the distance target is perfectly centered in the middle of the hole in the card, and lastly, moves the card toward his or her face, keeping the "E" target in the center of the hole. The dominant eye can be identified as the eye that the patient repeatedly uses at distance with the card. Another simple method requires the patient to hold a finger to create a hole in front of the two eyes horizontally at arm's length and gaze at a distant object through the hole (Figure 41-1). When the patient closes or occludes one eye, the dominant eye will be the one in which the image did not change; otherwise, this is the nondominant eye. One other method, though not commercially available in the United States, is described in a paper by Handa et al, in which they quantitatively measured ocular dominance using binocular rivalry induced by retinometers.[1]

Conclusion

Checking eye dominance is very important in a variety of clinical situations and should be checked prior to initiating any types of treatments or therapies.

References

1. Handa T, Uozato H, Higa R, et al. Quantitative measurement of ocular dominance using binocular rivalry induced by retinometers. *J Cataract Refract Surg.* 2006;32:831-836.
2. Jain S, Arora I, Azar DT. Success of monovision in presbyopes: Review of the literature and potential applications to refractive surgery. *Surv Ophthalmol.* 1996;40:491-499.

3. Tomita M, Kanamori T, Waring GO, et al. Simultaneous corneal inlay implantation and laser in situ keratomileusis for presbyopia in patients with hyperopia, myopia, or emmetropia: Six-month results. *J Cataract Refract Surg.* 2012;38:495-506.

4. Stahl JE. Conductive keratoplasty for presbyopia: 1-year results. *J Refract Surg.* 2006;22:137-144.

5. Goes FJ. Visual results following implantation of a refractive multifocal IOL in one eye and a diffractive multifocal IOL in the contralateral eye. *J Refract Surg.* 2008;24:300-305.

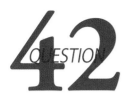

QUESTION 42

DO YOU CONSIDER PUPIL SIZE WHEN CHOOSING A PRESBYOPIA-CORRECTING IOL? WHY OR WHY NOT?

Roger F. Steinert, MD

Refractive surgeons typically are familiar with the concerns over pupil size and corneal laser refractive surgery. Although it seems intuitive that a patient will have optical disturbances when the edge of the entrance pupil expands beyond the edge of the laser ablation zone, careful study of patient outcomes has tended to refute this simple explanation for patient complaints about dim light vision.[1] Optical issues such as spherical aberration seem to be more important, as well as other perceptual psycho-physical variations between patients that are still poorly understood.

In contrast, although cataract surgeons occasionally experience patients with visual disturbances that cannot be explained, perhaps due to optical issues similar to those encountered in corneal refractive surgery, presbyopia-correcting intraocular lenses (IOLs) do have some specific optical issues clearly attributable to pupil size.

Accommodating-Design Intraocular Lenses

IOLs designed for presbyopia correction through accommodative mechanisms often have optical elements smaller than the typical 6.0-mm optical zone of standard IOLs. Smaller optical zones risk the occurrence of edge-related glare.

A case in point is the Bausch + Lomb Crystalens. The initial model, AT-45, had only a 4.5-mm optic diameter. Subsequent models have a 5.0-mm diameter. The potential for edge glare is increased, in addition to the smaller diameter itself, by the recommended surgical technique of having the capsulorrhexis margin larger than the optic, in the hope of allowing the optic to flex forward more readily when not restrained by the anterior capsule. A surgeon following this strategy does not have the potential benefit of edge glare reduction from an opacified anterior capsule overlying the edge of the IOL optic.

Henderson BA, Yoo SH. *Curbside Consultation in Refractive and Lens-Based Surgery: 49 Clinical Questions* (pp 171-173)
© 2015 SLACK Incorporated

A surgeon considering using this IOL or a similar smaller optic IOL should consider, therefore, whether the scotopic pupil enlarges beyond 5 mm. In the management of postoperative patient complaints suggestive of edge glare, the principal method of treatment is the use of miotic pharmaceuticals, typically brimonidine, or, if a stronger response is required, pilocarpine. Very weak concentrations such as 0.5% or 0.25% should be used at the beginning in order to build up tolerance.

Multifocal Intraocular Lenses

In most cases, multifocal IOLs have a 6.0-mm diameter, and the surgeon has the option of employing a smaller capsulorrhexis that will overlay the edge of the optic and reduce the potential of edge glare from a large scotopic pupil size.

However, different multifocal optic designs present different issues related to pupil size.

Refractive Optics Multifocal Intraocular Lenses

Both the original Array and the subsequent ReZoom IOL (Abbott Medical Optics) are based on refractive optics with a central optic that focuses for distance. With this lens design, a patient who has a very small (approximately 2 mm or less) pupil during near vision, perhaps made even smaller by a strong reading light, may lose the benefit of near optics and be unable to read.

Anticipating this scenario during a preoperative consultation is clinically challenging. No standard or readily applied method of measuring pupil size while reading is generally available or agreed upon, nor is the clinician in the office able to determine the patient's standard preferred level of illumination while reading at home. The best attempt at standardization may be the "Salzburg desk," but this is not available in most clinical environments.[2]

Postoperatively, diagnosis of excessive miosis while reading is generally done by administering a weak dilating agent such as phenylephrine 2.5%, and measuring reading vision before and after pupillary dilation to about 3 mm. Permanent increase in pupil size can be obtained by either photocoagulation of a circle of spots in the mid-iris or by creating several small sphincterotomies with the Nd:YAG laser.

Diffractive Optics Intraocular Lenses

Currently available diffractive optic IOLs present a different challenge related to pupil size. The principal complication with multifocal IOLs is halo and glare at night, and pupil size, combined with the diffractive optic design, interacts with the perception of halos and glare.

Halo and glare are largely attributable to the perception of the light from distance that passed through the near portion of the multifocal IOL. Distance light that passes through the near portion of the optic will focus in front of the retina and then diffuse. During the day, when the object and the surround tend to have the same illumination level, the diffused, lower energy "halo" light is not perceived. In contrast, at night, when a high-energy object (headlight, taillight, illuminated sign) is viewed, the surround is typically dark. Therefore, the out of focus "halo" light is perceived.

To try to reduce this problem, the Alcon ReSTOR IOL utilizes a strategy known as *apodization*. Basically, the ratio of distance to near focus increases as the optical zone increases. In theory, this should reduce complaints of night halo and glare. The downside, however, comes when a subject tries to read under dim light. If the pupil is large, the ability to read diminishes markedly.

Other manufacturers of diffractive multifocal IOLs (eg, the Abbott Medical Optics Tecnis IOLs) have designs that maintain a consistent ratio of distance and near focus over all pupil sizes, resulting in pupil size independence for distance and reading vision. Clinical studies have varied on whether the apodization strategy reduces night vision complaints and whether the compromise of dim light reading vision is a reasonable trade-off.[3]

If the main complaint is loss of reading vision with dim illumination with an apodized IOL, then the patient may benefit from a weak miotic pharmaceutical, as previously outlined, or by learning to carry a penlight to the restaurant. Often, the most satisfactory approach from the patient's standpoint is to use a different design multifocal IOL in the fellow eye.

Conclusion

Pupil size does have an impact on the performance and potential complications of many presbyopia-correcting IOLs. The absence of standard and widely available clinical measurements of pupil size under typical lifestyle conditions hampers a methodical approach to including the variable of pupil size in selecting an appropriate IOL for a patient. Understanding a patient's lifestyle and vision tasks is a guide for selecting a specific model of presbyopia IOL, and also helps suggest strategies to reduce postoperative issues raised by unhappy patients.

References

1. Chan A, Manche EE. Effect of preoperative pupil size on quality of vision after wavefront-guided LASIK. *Ophthalmology*. 2011;118:736-741.
2. Dexl AK. Application of the Salzburg reading desk in accommodation and presbyopic research. *Klin Monbl Augenheilkd*. 2011;228:676-680.
3. Rasp M, Bachernegg A, Seyeddain O, et al. Bilateral reading performance of 4 multifocal intraocular lens models and a monofocal intraocular lens under bright lighting conditions. *J Cataract Refract Surg*. 2012;38(11):1950-1961.

43

How Do You Center a Multifocal IOL, and Is It Important?

Richard Tipperman, MD

In order to answer this question, you must first ask yourself, what does it mean for an intraocular lens (IOL) to be centered? Although this rhetorical question seems simple, it is clear based on clinical observation that the answer must be complex.

I have seen patients with multifocal IOLs with rings "perfectly" centered referable to the pupil who were unhappy with their vision, while other patients whose rings were not centered were thrilled with their vision. These findings may seem confusing, until you realize that it may be wrong to view IOL centration with regard to pupillary geometry.

It is more important for a multifocal IOL to be centered referable to your patient's true visual axis rather than the geometric center of his or her pupil. In many patients, the visual axis will be close to the geometric center of the pupil, but in others it will be distant enough so that if the IOL is positioned on the geometric center of the visual axis, it will not be centered on the true visual axis.

Angle Kappa

The previous paragraph describes the visual optics principle of *angle kappa*. Although many describe angle kappa as the distance from the patient's true visual axis to the geometric center of the pupil, the true definition is that the angle kappa is the angular distance (in object space) between the line of sight and the pupillary axis[1] (Figure 43-1). The pupillary axis is the line perpendicular to the cornea that intersects the center of the entrance pupil.

Henderson BA, Yoo SH. *Curbside Consultation in Refractive and Lens-Based Surgery: 49 Clinical Questions* (pp 175-177)
© 2015 SLACK Incorporated

Figure 43-1. Schematic representation of angle kappa in relation to the line of sight. (Reprinted with permission from Pablo Artal blog [http://pabloartal.blogspot.com].)

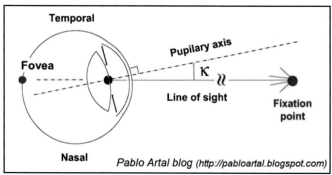

Angle kappa is important because if it is greater than half the diameter of the central optical zone of a multifocal IOL, the primary path of light may traverse one of the multifocal rings instead of the central optic, leading to glare or reduction in quality of vision.[2]

How Are Visual Axis and Angle Kappa Determined?

The visual axis, and therefore the angle kappa, can be determined in the office through a careful penlight examination. The patient can be asked to look at a penlight held in the distance and the separation of the light reflex from the geometric center of the visual can be measured. Although theoretically this may be a possibility, pragmatically, it is neither easily done nor quantitatively accurate. Several diagnostic devices allow for rapid, quantitative, and accurate measurement of angle kappa.

Although these measurements will assist you in preoperative planning, they still do not facilitate multifocal IOL centration at the time of surgery.

Ensuring Intraocular Lens Centration During Surgery

In many patients, the macula is displaced temporally and inferiorly with regard to a line drawn perpendicular to the geometric center of the pupil. As a result, the true visual axis will tend to be located nasally and superiorly to the geometric center of the pupil. To help with IOL centration, you can nudge the IOL slightly nasally and superiorly following completion of cataract surgery and removal of viscoelastic.

Although this approach may improve the accuracy of overall IOL centration, it does not individualize the geometry to the specific patient. A more individualized approach can be obtained by using either specific instrumentation designed for centration, or by using the coaxial light reflex from the operating microscope. Depending on the optics of the specific operating microscope, it may be possible to use the coaxial light illumination source to center the IOL. You should discuss the approach with a representative of the manufacturer of your specific operating microscope.

Another approach is to utilize an instrument set (eg, the Mastel Precision Centration Set). This consists of a pair of high magnification spectacles that have an LED light mounted on the nasal bridge. Instruct the patient to "look at the light on the bridge of my nose" and the high magnification spectacles allow you to see the light reflex of the LED on the cornea, clearly marking the "true" visual axis. You can then use a circular marker to make an impression on the corneal dome to aid with IOL centration at the conclusion of the surgery.

Conclusion

Work by Prakash et al has demonstrated that significant IOL decentration can lead to optical distortion, photic phenomenon, and reduction of quality of vision.[2] Measurement of angle kappa can be performed preoperatively to aid in your surgical decision making. You then have a variety of options available to aid in IOL centration at the time of surgery.

References

1. On the definition of angle kappa. Available at: http://pabloartal.blogspot.com/2008/08/on-definition-of-angle-kappa.html. Retrieved on April 8, 2014.
2. Prakash G, Prakash DR, Agarwal A, Kumar DA, Agarwal A, Jacob S. Predictive factor and kappa angle analysis for visual satisfactions in patients with multifocal IOL implantation. *Eye*. 2011;25(9):1187-1193.

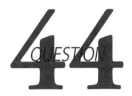

HOW DO YOU MANAGE AN UNHAPPY MULTIFOCAL PATIENT WHO IS EXPERIENCING HALOS AND GLARE?

Laura Vickers, MD and Terry Kim, MD

Patients with multifocal intraocular lenses (IOLs) have complained of symptoms including blurry vision, photic phenomena such as glare and halos, negative dysphotopsia, and "ghosting" of images.[1] Some studies have described patient experiences of decreased contrast sensitivity, decreased visual acuity at certain working distances, and increased intraocular stray light.[2] Glare and halos may occur in about 30% of patients with multifocal IOLs.[2-4] Although patients with monofocal lenses may also experience dysphotopsia, there is a trend toward more noticeable and larger halos in patients with multifocal lenses. Dysphotopsia can result from simultaneous projection of multiple images by the IOL, and in most cases, patients adapt well within the first few months. However, this phenomenon can be amplified by multiple additional factors.

The first step we take in addressing any kind of patient dissatisfaction after surgery is attentive listening and reassurance. With a systematic approach, we label "the six Cs." Most causes of suboptimal vision with multifocal lenses can be readily addressed with resulting patient satisfaction. Preserving patient confidence requires an empathetic approach; knowing what steps to take next is crucial for any surgeon using multifocal IOLs in his or her practice.

1. The first C is for *cornea*—causes relating to dry eyes, anterior basement membrane dystrophy, Salzmann's nodular degeneration, Fuchs' endothelial dystrophy, and other corneal pathology. Dry eye, blepharitis, and meibomian gland dysfunction are common causes of blurry vision in this setting, and should be treated appropriately with artificial tears and ointments, warm compresses, and lid hygiene *before* surgery to avoid such complaints later. Prior to surgery, visually significant anterior basement membrane dystrophy and Salzmann's nodules should be treated with epithelial debridement and/or superficial keratectomy and repeat keratometry and biometry performed at least 1 month after the ocular surface has healed for more accurate IOL calculation (Figure 44-1). Careful corneal examination, along with pachymetry and

Henderson BA, Yoo SH. *Curbside Consultation in Refractive and Lens-Based Surgery: 49 Clinical Questions* (pp 179-181)
© 2015 SLACK Incorporated

Figure 44-1. Central anterior basement membrane dystrophy. (A) Slit-lamp photographs demonstrating central corneal changes under diffuse illumination and red reflex. (B) Corresponding corneal topography of the same eye. (C) Corneal topography after treatment with epithelial debridement. (Reprinted with permission from David T. Vroman, MD.)

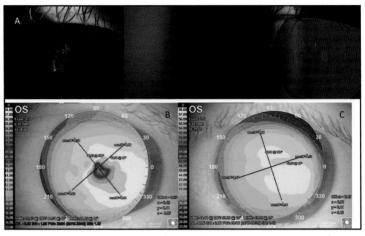

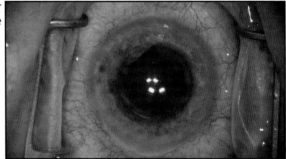

Figure 44-2. Centering a ReSTOR intraocular lens implant using Purkinje images from the operating room microscope light reflex.

specular microscopy, may be useful in identifying patients with moderate to severe guttata or frank Fuchs' dystrophy, which we view as relative contraindications for multifocal IOL implantation. Due to several reasons (unpredictable hyperopic refractive shift, induced astigmatism, higher-order aberrations),[5] patients who have received or may require full or partial-thickness corneal transplantation are not candidates for multifocal IOL surgery.

2. The second C is for *cylinder*, or residual refractive error. Patients are most commonly bothered by astigmatism, but also by residual spherical myopia or hyperopia. The most common cause of patient dissatisfaction after placement of a multifocal lens in one prospective study was anisometropia and astigmatism, making up almost 65% of cases.[1] These cases can be addressed with spectacles, contact lenses, limbal relaxing incision/astigmatic keratotomy, or photorefractive keratectomy/LASIK.

3. The third C is for *centration*. IOL decentration can result from retention of cortical/lens material, IOL rotation, and capsular contraction, among other causes. In an effort to optimize multifocal IOL centration intraoperatively, we try to align the center ring of the multifocal IOL with the Purkinje images of the operating microscope light while the patient is asked to fixate on the center of the light (Figure 44-2). Postoperatively, we examine the patient to ensure that the center ring of the multifocal IOL is centered with respect to the undilated pupil. In general, mild decentration of the multifocal IOL does not seem to adversely affect vision. However, moderate to severe decentration can affect quality of vision. In these instances, we recommend first trying an argon laser iridoplasty using Dr. Eric Donnenfeld's technique where argon laser spots (500-micron spot size, 500 mW, 500-millisecond duration with appropriate titration based on iris color) are placed in the mid-peripheral iris in the direc-

tion in which you wish the pupil edge to move. If this proves unsuccessful, the patient may have to return to the operating room to address the underlying reason for IOL decentration and/or IOL repositioning. We then use the Purkinje images of the light microscope to help realign the IOL. In our experience, most patients tolerate small amounts of decentration.

4. The fourth C is for *capsule*. Careful inspection of the posterior capsule is merited because a large proportion of blurry vision and photic complaints with multifocal IOLs are related to subtle posterior capsular opacification or wrinkling, which can be addressed with YAG laser posterior capsulotomy at least 1 month after surgery.

5. The fifth C is for *cystoid macular edema* and other retinal issues including diabetic retinopathy, epiretinal membrane, and age-related macular degeneration, which we view as relative contraindications to multifocal IOL selection. The importance of screening for these conditions before considering a multifocal IOL cannot be overemphasized, as any macular pathology can magnify the effects associated with multifocal IOLs, especially glare, halos, and decreased contrast sensitivity. Prescreening retinal optical coherence tomography (OCT) imaging and prophylactic treatment with topical nonsteroidal anti-inflammatory drug therapy are worthwhile in these multifocal IOL candidates prior to surgery.

6. The sixth and final C is for *cerebral*. Occasionally, patients are simply intolerant of the multifocal IOL. Photic phenomena comprise the most common complaint that remains unexplained by objective findings on examination. While acuity may be improved to 20/20, some patients will continue to describe symptoms of intolerable glare and halos, "waxy vision," or decreased contrast sensitivity. In these patients, an IOL exchange for a monofocal IOL may be required. Ideally, careful patient selection will help to avoid these cases.

All patients should be counseled on the potential limitations and side effects of multifocal IOL selection. One of the most important aspects of the face-to-face patient encounter is to determine if the patient has realistic expectations with respect to the procedure. Patients who may be at higher risk for experiencing these postoperative problems or those with unrealistic expectations are probably not ideal candidates for multifocal IOLs.

References

1. de Vries NE, Webers CA, Touwslager WR, et al. Dissatisfaction after implantation of multifocal intraocular lenses. *J Cataract Refract Surg*. 2011;37(5):859-865.
2. Souza CE, Muccioli C, Soriano ES, et al. Visual performance of AcrySof ReSTOR apodized diffractive IOL: A prospective comparative trial. *Am J Ophthalmol*. 2006;141(5):827-832.
3. Sen HN, Sarikkola AU, Uusitalo RJ, Laatikainen L. Quality of vision after AMO Array multifocal intraocular lens implantation. *J Cataract Refract Surg*. 2004;30(12):2483-2493.
4. Zhao G, Zhang J, Zhou Y, et al. Visual function after monocular implantation of apodized diffractive multifocal or single-piece monofocal intraocular lens: Randomized prospective comparison. *J Cataract Refract Surg*. 2010;36(2):282-285.
5. Lichtinger A, Yeung SN, Kim T. Top 5 pearls to consider when implanting advanced-technology IOLs in patients with a compromised cornea. *Int Ophthalmol Clin*. 2012;52(2):59-63.

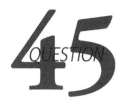

WHEN SHOULD THE POSTERIOR CAPSULE BE OPENED WITH A YAG? DO YOU DO IT SOONER RATHER THAN LATER, OR WAIT UNTIL THE LAST MOMENT?

Mark Packer, MD, FACS, CPI

I base my approach to YAG capsulotomy on the patient's subjective quality of vision, clinical tests such as visual acuity and brightness acuity, the patient's degree of desire for spectacle independence, and the type and status of the intraocular lens (IOL). It is a very different calculus when considering a patient with a monofocal IOL who doesn't mind wearing glasses vs a patient with a refractive IOL (toric, accommodative, or multifocal) who has an expressed desire for spectacle freedom. In addition, decentration, tilt, or malposition of the IOL may play a role in the decision making.

For a patient wearing bifocal glasses with an aspheric or spherical monofocal IOL in good position, I wouldn't really consider a YAG until the patient is symptomatic from posterior capsular opacification (PCO). By far, the most common symptom of PCO is decreased night vision with glare, and it is best documented clinically with a Brightness Acuity Test (BAT). Incidentally, Medicare carriers and other payers in the United States generally base their criteria for the appropriateness of YAG capsulotomy on BAT visual acuity with the medium brightness setting (generally a loss of two lines from best-corrected visual acuity qualifies).

Because glare symptoms can also result from decentration or tilt of an IOL, in some cases, a repositioning procedure would be indicated rather than a YAG. An IOL should be well-centered, usually with 360-degree overlap of the anterior capsule on the optic. Repositioning is significantly safer and easier to perform in the presence of an intact capsule prior to YAG capsulotomy. In this regard, it is also critical to differentiate lens-related dysphotopsia from the visual effects of PCO. The classic "temporal crescent" of negative dysphotopsia may be better treated with a piggyback IOL.[1]

Henderson BA, Yoo SH. *Curbside Consultation in Refractive and Lens-Based Surgery: 49 Clinical Questions* (pp 183-188)
© 2015 SLACK Incorporated

With refractive IOLs (toric, multifocal, and accommodative), it is worth considering the refractive effect of the YAG capsulotomy, especially in those cases pending a possible enhancement procedure. Yilmaz et al found a mean change in manifest spherical equivalent refraction of 0.22 to 0.38 diopters (D) following YAG,[2] while Vrijman et al found a change in spherical equivalent of greater than 0.5 D in 7% of eyes.[3] If a refractive procedure is contemplated for residual pseudophakic refractive error and there is an indication of progressive PCO, it makes sense to advance the capsulotomy so that any potential additional change in refractive error can be corrected at the same time. If, however, the posterior capsule is pristine, the IOL has a 360-degree posterior square edge, the capsulorrhexis completely overlaps the optic, and there are no other reasons to anticipate the development of symptomatic PCO, I don't think it's necessary to YAG first. Also, I would not generally YAG prior to inserting a piggyback IOL to correct residual refractive error (or dysphotopsia). The potential for vitreous entanglement or IOL dislocation is too great.

Multifocal IOLs carry a special caution with regard to YAG capsulotomy because of the combined one-two punch of multifocal dysphotopsia and the risks of IOL exchange after YAG. Halos around lights at night, glare, and a host of other unique aberrations may accompany the implantation of multifocal IOLs. Multifocal IOLs can be extraordinarily successful for many patients, and, in fact, the satisfaction rate (ie, percent of patients who would choose the same IOL again) is about 95%. Nevertheless, a small percentage of people are extremely bothered by multifocal dysphotopsia, even to the point of desiring IOL exchange. The situation becomes more complex when there is PCO, because then a decision must be made: exchange or YAG? Once the YAG is performed, the risks of an IOL exchange rise due to the likelihood of vitreous prolapse and subsequent retinal complications.

Before taking action, you must determine the etiology of the dysphotopsia: is it primarily due to the IOL or the capsule? One way to help untangle this knot is to ask whether the symptoms have been present ever since the IOL was implanted, or increased gradually after implantation (usually PCO is not present in the immediate postoperative period). Other helpful indicators include the nature of the dysphotopsia (pure halos are more likely IOL-related) and the visual acuity (PCO generally degrades acuity, but multifocal dysphotopsia often coexists with excellent acuity). BAT is not generally helpful in these cases. It is also worth considering that proliferative PCO can be polished from the capsule during an exchange. Anecdotally, I have exchanged an older type of refractive multifocal IOL for a newer diffractive model while cleaning the capsule in the same procedure, resulting in a very happy patient.

Another special case exists for accommodative IOLs, in particular the Crystalens (Bausch + Lomb). This lens is designed with hinged haptics, and may undergo more extreme variations of positioning than single or three-piece IOLs due to capsular contraction (Figures 45-1 and 45-2).[4] YAG capsulotomy is often the treatment of choice for Z-syndrome. In addition, YAG may result in greater effects on the refractive spherical equivalent following YAG. Therefore, the caveat about refractive IOLs applies even more strongly to the Crystalens: if there is any indication of progressive PCO or capsular contraction in a patient desiring keratorefractive enhancement, do YAG first.

I do have a concern about dislocation of certain IOLs after YAG. There are still a few plate haptic silicone IOLs around, and the force of capsular contraction is known to squeeze these IOLs into the vitreous cavity following YAG. Make a small capsulotomy and warn the patient about sudden loss of vision. A similar warning applies to dual optic accommodative IOLs, such as the Synchrony (Abbott Medical Optics), although these lenses have an extraordinarily low rate of PCO.

As you can see, I prefer a personalized approach to YAG based on the patient's refractive goals and the status of the IOL. Making these types of decisions is at the heart of refractive lens surgery.

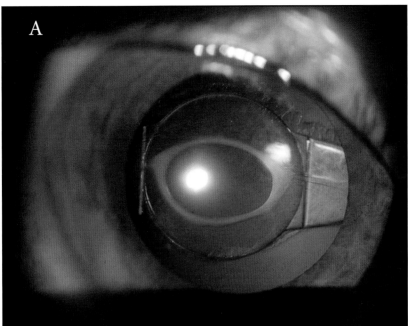

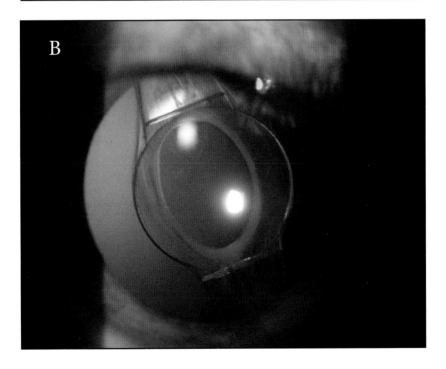

Figure 45-1. (A and B) A 48-year-old woman with high myopia and astigmatism underwent refractive lens exchange with an accommodative IOL (Crystalens AT-45, Bausch + Lomb). Six weeks postoperatively, she developed decreased best-corrected visual acuity and slit-lamp examination demonstrated bilateral anterior capsular phimosis. *(continued)*

**Figure   45-1
(continued).** (C
and D) The mani-
fest   refractive
spherical equiva-
lent (MRSE) mea-
sured Plano OD
and   +0.125 OS.
Anterior segment
optical   coher-
ence   tomogra-
phy   (AS-OCT,
Visante, Carl Zeiss
Meditec) demon-
strated an anteri-
or chamber depth
(ACD) of 7.06 mm
OD and 6.04 mm
OS.

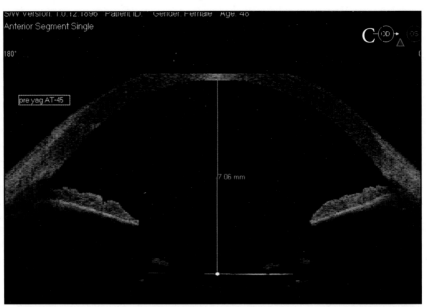

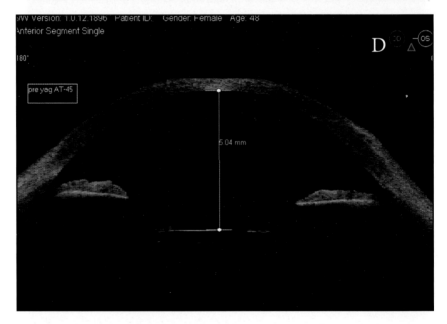

References

1. Masket S, Fram NR. Pseudophakic negative dysphotopsia: Surgical management and new theory of etiology. *J Cataract Refract Surg.* 2011;37(7):1199-1207.
2. Yilmaz S, Ozdil MA, Bozkir N, Maden A. The effect of Nd:YAG laser capsulotomy size on refraction and visual acuity. *J Refract Surg.* 2006;22(7):719-721.
3. Vrijman V, van der Linden JW, Nieuwendaal CP, van der Meulen IJ, Mourits MP, Lapid-Gortzak R. Effect of Nd:YAG laser capsulotomy on refraction in multifocal apodized diffractive pseudophakia. *J Refract Surg.* 2012;28(8):545-550.
4. Yuen L, Trattler W, Boxer Wachler BS. Two cases of Z syndrome with the Crystalens after uneventful cataract surgery. *J Cataract Refract Surg.* 2008;34(11):1986-1989.

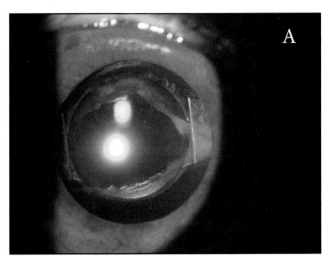

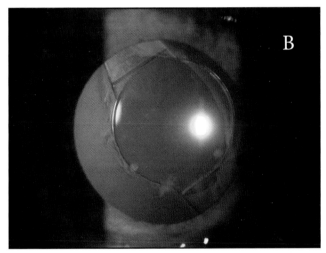

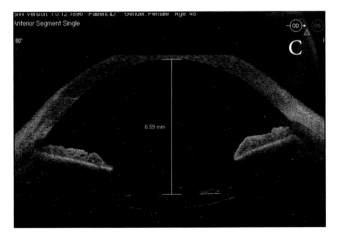

Figure 45-2. (A and B) Following anterior YAG relaxing capsulotomy OU the visual acuity improved. The slit-lamp appearance showed resolution of the phimosis. (C) AS-OCT demonstrated an *anterior* shift of the IOL in the right eye, resulting in a more myopic MRSE (Δ ACD OD = 6.59 – 7.06 = –0.47 mm anterior shift of +10.75 D IOL 0.125 D refractive shift). *(continued)*

Figure 45-2 (continued). (D) In the left eye, AS-OCT revealed a posterior shift of the IOL, resulting in a more hyperopic MRSE (Δ ACD OS = 6.51 − 5.04 = 1.47 mm posterior shift of +11.50 D IOL + 0.250 D shift refractive shift). The patient ultimately underwent LASIK OU to correct the residual refractive error.

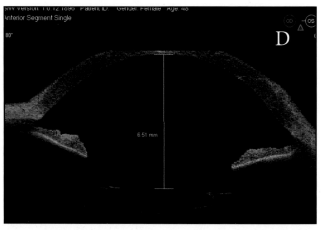

HOW WOULD YOU TREAT A +1.50 D RESIDUAL REFRACTIVE ERROR IN A PATIENT WITH A MULTIFOCAL IOL? HOW ABOUT −1.00 D? HOW ABOUT +1.25 D ASTIGMATISM?

Hiroko Bissen-Miyajima, MD, PhD

Refractive error following the implantation of a multifocal intraocular lens (IOL) is usually an unexpected surprise for both the ophthalmologist and the patient. The patient who chooses the multifocal IOL wants spectacle independence and requires good uncorrected distance and near visual acuities. The residual refractive error of +1.5 diopters (D) or −1.00 D would definitely decrease the uncorrected visual acuity and the patient would not be satisfied with the surgical outcome.

As for refractive error following the implantation of a multifocal IOL, I consider the treatment in 3 steps:

1. Ask the patient if she or he wishes for better vision or to maintain the vision as it is. To my surprise, some patients are happy despite the residual refractive error.

2. Let the patient experience the improved vision by testing lenses with spherical and cylindrical correction. By testing lenses, the patient can approximate the improved visual acuity after the treatment. At this time, the patient should also consider the difference of vision at distance, intermediate, and near. Even distance vision improves with the testing lens, and some patients place an importance on both near and intermediate vision without the testing lens.

3. If the correction of residual refractive error is planned, the simultaneous bilateral or unilateral procedure should be considered. In case of a similar amount of residual refractive error in both eyes, bilateral treatment may be a good choice. If there are some differences in the amount of the refractive error, I prefer to treat the eye with the larger amount of the error at first and see the improvement of the vision. In my experience, some patients are happy with unilateral correction and do not want the fellow eye to be treated. The reason is that the eye that has some refractive error shows the benefit of depth of focus.

Henderson BA, Yoo SH. *Curbside Consultation in Refractive and Lens-Based Surgery: 49 Clinical Questions* (pp 189-191)
© 2015 SLACK Incorporated

Figure 46-1. Contrast sensitivity measured by CSV-1000 in eyes with multifocal IOLs. There was no significant change between before and after wavefront-guided LASIK (paired t-test).

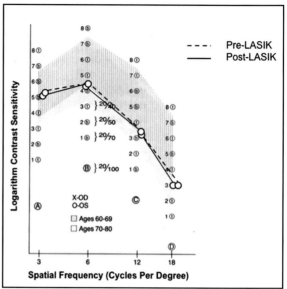

In addition to the previous 3 steps, we should keep in mind the possible changes of residual refraction, especially the cylindrical change over the long term. The shift to against-the-rule astigmatism following cataract surgery has been reported.[1] In the case of +1.25 D astigmatism, the amount of treatment differs depending on the axis of the astigmatism. Against-the-rule astigmatism should be fully corrected; however, with-the-rule astigmatism should be aimed slightly under the correction.

Next, we need to consider the surgical procedure. Since most refractive error is a combination of spherical and cylindrical, my first choice of correction is LASIK using the femtosecond laser. The excellent surgical outcomes of LASIK have been reported in eyes following the implantation of multifocal IOLs.[2-4] The use of wavefront technology in excimer laser treatment has been discussed. When I can confirm that Shack-Hartmann aberrometers measured the distance correction, I usually perform wavefront-guided LASIK. In cases of astigmatism, the iris registration is very helpful to determine the axis of astigmatism. Excellent predictability and surgical outcomes have been reported. In my series of 43 eyes, contrast sensitivity in eyes with the multifocal IOL did not change after the refractive correction with LASIK (Figure 46-1). I believe the amount of ablation is smaller than most LASIK cases and does not influence the visual quality. Laser arcuate incision is becoming popular. Although the nomogram of arcuate keratotomy with the femtosecond laser is improved, the predictability of astigmatic correction is superior in LASIK in my experience. Also, LASIK has the advantage of treating not only the astigmatism, but also the spherical error.

My answer for the treatment of +1.5, −1.00, or +1.25 D astigmatism is simple when I consider LASIK if the patient wishes for better uncorrected visual acuity. If the eye ended up with the residual refraction of +1.5 D, the patient cannot benefit from the multifocal IOL for both distance and near, and full correction with LASIK shows promising results. If the residual refractive error is −1.00 D, some patients are happy with good near and intermediate visual acuities. If both eyes have similar refractive errors, I would probably perform unilateral correction. I will double-check the bilateral vision while leaving the fellow eye myopic, or the fellow eye corrected with a trial lens of −1.00 D. I have had some patients who enjoyed good visual acuity at all distances with one emmetropic eye and slight myopia in the fellow eye. The treatment of astigmatism of +1.25 D is more complicated than that of spherical error. As I mentioned before, the amount of the correction should be considered according to the axis of the astigmatism. In most astigmatic cases, the additional spherical correction with LASIK is mandatory.

References

1. Hayashi K, Hirata A, Manabe S, Hayashi H. Long-term change in corneal astigmatism after sutureless cataract surgery. *Am J Ophthalmol.* 2011;151:858-865.
2. Jendritza BB, Knorz MC, Morton S. Wavefront-guided excimer laser vision correction after multifocal IOL implantation. *J Refract Surg.* 2008;24:274-279.
3. Alfonso JF, Fernández-vega L, Montés-micó R, Valcárcel B. Femtosecond laser for residual refractive error correction after refractive lens exchange with multifocal intraocular lens implantation. *Am J Ophthalmol.* 2008;146:244-250.
4. Muftuoglu O, Prasher P, Chu C, et al. Laser in situ keratomileusis for residual refractive errors after apodized diffractive multifocal intraocular lens implantation. *J Cataract Refract Surg.* 2009;35:1063-1071.

AFTER IMPLANTATION OF AN ACCOMMODATING IOL, HOW WOULD YOU TREAT –1.5-D RESIDUAL REFRACTIVE ERROR, 1.5-D WITH-THE-RULE ASTIGMATIC ERROR, AND 1.5-D AGAINST-THE-RULE ASTIGMATIC ERROR?

Parag Parekh, MD, MPA and Louis D. "Skip" Nichamin, MD

–1.5-D Residual Refractive Error

For any of these situations, usually the first step is to determine why the residual refractive error exists.

Was there a history of refractive surgery (LASIK, photorefractive keratectomy [PRK])? Using standard intraocular lens (IOL) calculation techniques, previous myopic LASIK/PRK typically results in a hyperopic surprise after cataract surgery, while prior hyperopic LASIK/PRK generally leads to a myopic surprise (though less so because the central corneal power is less affected by a hyperopic LASIK/PRK treatment). Previous radial keratotomy can lead to corneal instability, irregular astigmatism, and hyperopic shift over time. If the cornea was stable prior to cataract surgery, it is likely to remain stable postoperatively, after some initial postoperative fluctuation.

Were the IOL calculations imprecise because of dry eye, epithelial basement membrane dystrophy (EBMD), or technician error? Ocular surface issues can play an important role in refractive surprises. It is important to address these conditions prior to IOL calculation with proper treatment of dry eye, blepharitis, and other surface issues. In cases of significant EBMD, Salzmann's degeneration, or similar conditions, we will frequently perform phototherapeutic keratectomy (PTK) first and then proceed with IOL calculations after the epithelium has healed and the ocular surface is optimized.

Is the IOL malpositioned? Accommodating IOLs have flexible haptics and are meant to be placed in a posterior-vault configuration. On slit-lamp examination, one needs to determine if the IOL is properly vaulted, with the plane of the optic posterior to that of the haptics. An

Henderson BA, Yoo SH. *Curbside Consultation in Refractive and Lens-Based Surgery: 49 Clinical Questions* (pp 193-194) © 2015 SLACK Incorporated

anterior-vault configuration could explain a myopic result. This can be caused by a capsular distention-type syndrome, or possibly by exuberant capsular phimosis and contraction, or malpositioned haptics. In this case, one may have to use a YAG laser, or less likely, surgically reopen the bag, rotate the IOL 90 degrees, and consider placing a capsular tension ring to re-establish the proper posterior vault.

Once the source of the error is understood, the ocular surface has been optimized, and the IOL is confirmed to be in good position, we suggest YAG capsulotomy prior to a refractive enhancement. There can sometimes be a refractive shift after the capsulotomy and one needs to know the final amount of stable refractive error that will require treatment, and an open capsule will permit the best and most accurate refraction prior to refractive correction.

Next, in most cases we suggest an excimer laser enhancement, usually PRK, to treat the residual refractive error. If there was a distinct contraindication for a laser keratorefractive procedure, another solution is to place a sulcus "piggyback" IOL to treat the residual error. This latter option is particularly attractive when the posterior capsule is still intact, and corneal issues prevail.

One final consideration is to test whether the patient can tolerate monovision. One can get a sense of this by using a contact lens to bring the contralateral eye to plano. Alternatively, one might consider proceeding with cataract surgery in the contralateral eye, aiming for plano, and subsequently reassessing the patient's level of satisfaction. If inadequate, one can proceed with a laser enhancement or piggyback IOL for the original eye to bring it to plano.

1.5-D With-the-Rule Astigmatic Error and 1.5-D Against-the-Rule Astigmatic Error

For residual astigmatism, some investigation into the cause is again the first step. As noted above, the ocular surface must be optimized first.

Do the keratometry measurements and the topographic corneal astigmatism correspond to the measured astigmatism, or could the IOL be tilted? It is important to know the source of the residual astigmatism. For an accommodating IOL, one must determine whether the IOL has tilted, or is assuming a "Z" configuration. In these cases, one can use the YAG laser to release asymmetric capsular forces, or one may be required to surgically reopen the bag, rotate the IOL 90 degrees, and possibly place a capsular tension ring to re-establish the proper posterior vault. The status of the posterior capsule is always an important consideration when contemplating reentering the eye.

Was a limbal relaxing incision (LRI) performed concurrently with the cataract surgery, and does the residual astigmatic error represent either over- or undercorrection? In the case of an LRI that undercorrected the astigmatism, it is fairly straightforward to extend or re-deepen the original LRI. In the case of LRI overcorrection, we suggest an excimer laser ablation to correct the refractive error.

In cases where the spherical equivalent is close to plano, an LRI is probably the simplest way to treat the residual astigmatism. If there is a significant spherical component to the residual error, then excimer laser ablation is the preferred method of treatment. Of note, in other countries there are low-power toric piggyback IOLs available that could also be used in this situation.

Finally, in cases of against-the-rule astigmatic error, one might consider undercorrecting the error, leaving some of the against-the-rule astigmatism intact. This is thought to create a type of multifocality that can improve a patient's near vision, without excessive impairing of his or her distance vision.

48

WHAT CAUSES A Z-SYNDROME? HOW DO YOU DIAGNOSE AND MANAGE IT?

Peter A. Rapoza, MD, FACS

Intraocular lens (IOL) decentration and tilt have been issues since posterior chamber intraocular lenses (PC-IOLs) were introduced.[1] Irregularly centered anterior capsular openings with jagged edges made it difficult to ensure in-the-bag placement of both haptics. IOL rotation or dislocation from in-the-bag placement could result in one haptic in the bag and one in the sulcus. Capsular fibrosis could result in decentration of the optic and rotation around the long axis of the implant with tilt.

The safety and efficacy of cataract surgery is predicated on the successful creation of a well-centered continuous curvilinear capsulotomy, which allows (1) the surgeon to use a fluid wave to separate the cortex from the remaining capsule; (2) easy rotation of the lens cortex and nucleus within the capsular bag; and (3) a means of securing the PC-IOL in the sulcus if the posterior capsule is damaged, making in-the-bag placement of the haptics suboptimal.

Implantation of the original Ionics AT 45 Crystalens (Bausch+Lomb) was heralded as a significant advance. Although many Crystalens patients did report improvement in distance and intermediate visual acuities, the relatively small diameter optics were prone to decentration. Ophthalmologists noticed occasional cases of induction of myopia with astigmatism along the long axis of the IOL associated with anterior movement of one haptic, which, when associated with posterior movement of the other haptic, could deform the IOL into a "Z" shape when viewed from the side, thus the name "Z-syndrome."[2] The alteration in IOL position from that initially obtained postoperatively is due to posterior capsular contracture syndrome (PCCS). There exists a wide range of IOL shape alterations, from the desired posteriorly vaulted position where both haptics angle anteriorly and the optic is centered around and perpendicular to the visual axis, to a slight decrease in anterior angulation of one haptic beginning to tilt the optic posteriorly (Figure 48-1) to the true Z-syndrome as described previously (Figure 48-2). Even the Crystalens AO has been implicated.[3]

Henderson BA, Yoo SH. *Curbside Consultation in Refractive and Lens-Based Surgery: 49 Clinical Questions* (pp 195-198) © 2015 SLACK Incorporated

Figure 48-1. Crystalens AO with lens tilt. (Reprinted with permission from Bausch+Lomb.)

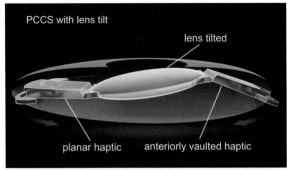

Figure 48-2. Crystalens AO with Z-syndrome. (Reprinted with permission from Bausch+Lomb.)

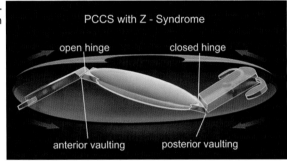

The treatment of Z-syndrome is dependent on the anatomic features present. Implants that failed to have both haptics implanted in the capsular bag immediately demonstrate a myopic shift with astigmatism in the long axis of the IOL. The definitive treatment of this variant begins with filling the anterior chamber and capsular bag with viscoelastic. Using a bimanual approach, a spatula keeps the optic in close apposition with the posterior capsule, while a Y-hook pushes the haptic that is out of the bag centrally and posteriorly to capture the haptic and footplates in the bag. The IOL is rotated 180 degrees to ensure that the haptics are at the equator. The phacoemulsification wound is prepared for closure with a preplaced 10-0 nylon suture and the viscoelastic removed by irrigation/aspiration, maintaining gentle pressure on the central portion of the optic and squeezing viscoelastic from between the posterior surface of the IOL and the posterior capsule. The suture is tied and balanced saline solution (BSS) irrigates through the paracentesis site behind the IOL to assure that all residual viscoelastic is removed. The planned position of the haptics is achieved and the Z-syndrome is resolved.

More frequently, the IOL is positioned with both haptics in the capsular bag and a normally positioned IOL is present at postoperative day 1, with the targeted refraction achieved. Within days, a myopic shift is noted associated with the appearance of astigmatism along the long axis of the IOL, which does not correlate with corneal astigmatism. These changes are associated with fibrosis in the peripheral capsular bag where the remaining anterior capsule and the underlying posterior capsule come into apposition, causing the haptic to lose posterior angulation. If the dilated examination reveals that the anterior capsular opening is not well centered and the tilt is along the axis of decentration, the anterior chamber and capsular bag are filled with viscoelastic to separate the capsular adhesions. The implant is then rotated so that the short axis of the implant is perpendicular to the axis of capsular opening decentration. If the capsular opening is relatively well centered around the optic, the situation can be addressed by use of selective and sometimes multiple incisions in the posterior capsule. The technique of selective capsular openings to relieve Crystalens tilt or a true Z-syndrome have been well described in a guide produced

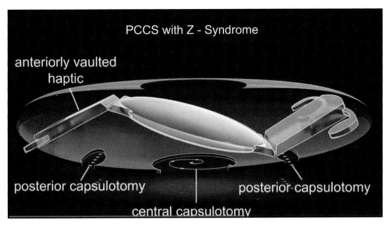

Figure 48-3. YAG laser treatment of Z-syndrome with multiple selective posterior capsulotomies (side view). (Reprinted with permission from Bausch + Lomb.)

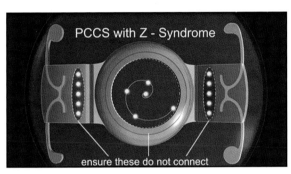

Figure 48-4. YAG laser treatment of Z-syndrome with multiple selective posterior capsulotomies (top view). (Reprinted with permission from Bausch + Lomb.)

by Bausch + Lomb in association with Harvey Carter, MD.[4] Prior to embarking on this approach, it is imperative that the surgeon confirm that both haptics are in the capsular bag because reposition of haptics once the capsule has been opened is difficult at best, and may lead to loss of adequate capsular support for the implant. YAG laser correction of implant tilt or Z-syndrome is best performed with a widely dilated pupil that gives the surgeon an unhindered view of the optic, the hinges, and the haptics. The initial slit-like incision tangential to the optic is placed beneath the anteriorly displaced haptic in an effort to use the "spring" action of the accommodating IOL to reposition the optic more perpendicular to the visual axis (Figures 48-3 and 48-4). If no significant change occurs, a second capsulotomy is performed centrally, taking care not to connect the initial slit incision with the usually larger circular opening. A final slit-like incision similar to the initial one can be placed beneath the posteriorly angled haptic, avoiding connection to the central posterior capsulotomy to try to give the implant more of an ability to flex into the desired posteriorly vaulted position. I have used this technique with success in eyes with mild tilt to frank Z-syndrome. In one eye, the laser technique did not fully correct the IOL positioning, so I used a cannula with a cohesive viscoelastic to separate the adhesions between the anterior and posterior capsules, returning the IOL to a posteriorly vaulted configuration and correcting the induced astigmatism. One can consider the addition of a capsular tension ring to discourage the apposition of the anterior and posterior capsules, either routinely or during intraoperative treatment of Z-syndrome eyes. Once the implant has been returned to a posteriorly vaulted position, stable residual astigmatism induced by the IOL can be treated by excimer laser ablation. If these maneuvers fail, consider IOL exchange, carefully removing the Crystalens and implanting a three-piece sulcus fixated PC-IOL in front of the capsular remnants.

Conclusion

Tilt or frank Z-syndrome appears to be much less frequent with the current generation of Crystalens. The best treatment is prevention by creating a well-centered anterior capsular opening of approximately 5-mm diameter, using BSS to effectively separate the cortex from the capsule, carefully removing all cortical material by a meticulous irrigation/aspiration clean-up, polishing the posterior capsule mechanically or via "power washing" the capsule with BSS. IOLs should be placed securely in the capsular bag with intraoperative confirmation in all cases. If capsulotomies are decentered, the IOL should be rotated appropriately so that the decentered zone is 90 degrees perpendicular to the long axis of the implant. Placement of a suture in the phacoemulsification incision and (if desired) in the paracentesis site reduces the risk of loss of chamber and movement of the IOL. Patients should be apprised that this uncommon syndrome may occur and that its rectification may require multiple steps to optimize the visual result.

References

1. Ale JB. Intraocular lens tilt and decentration: A concern for contemporary IOL designs. *Nepal J Ophthalmol.* 2011;3(5):68-77.
2. Cazal J, Lapine-Dapena C, Marín J, Vergés C. Accommodative intraocular lens tilting. *Am J Ophthalmol.* 2005;140:341-344.
3. Yuen L, Trattler W, Boxer Wachler BS. Two cases of Z syndrome with Crystalens after uneventful cataract surgery. *J Cataract Refract Surg.* 2008;34:1986-1989.
4. Clinical Pearls: YAG Treatment for Crystalens Patients. Bausch + Lomb Incorporated; 2009.

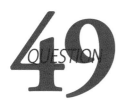

If the Implantation of an Accommodating IOL in the First Eye Did Not Yield Sufficient Uncorrected Near Vision, What Do You Recommend for the Second Eye?

Richard S. Hoffman, MD

Before deciding to implant either an accommodative or multifocal implant in a cataract or refractive lens exchange patient, a thorough discussion regarding potential limitations and side effects of the various intraocular lens (IOL) options should transpire. In my experience, a patient who strongly desires spectacle independence is a better candidate for a multifocal IOL rather than currently available single optic accommodative IOLs.[1] However, multifocal IOLs have potential optical aberrations, such as glare and halos, and are not good options for patients with corneal or macular pathology or patients with demanding, type A personalities.

If I implant a multifocal IOL in a patient, I will usually start with the nondominant eye. In this way, if patients are unhappy with the optical aberrations of multifocality, a monofocal or accommodative IOL in their dominant eye may ultimately work for them. The monofocal IOL gives the best possible visual quality in the dominant eye, while the multifocal IOL yields near vision with less distraction from the aberrations because they are present in the nondominant eye only. If patients are still unhappy with the multifocal IOL, an IOL exchange can be performed with a standard monofocal IOL or an accommodative IOL.

If I implant an accommodative IOL as my first choice, I will usually start with the dominant eye. In this way, if the patient does not achieve acceptable near vision, implantation for the second nondominant eye can be altered in order to maximize intermediate or near vision. There are perhaps three or four options for treating the second eye when a patient does not achieve adequate near vision from the first eye after accommodative IOL implantation.

When an accommodative IOL does not give adequate near vision, the cheapest option for the patient is implantation of a standard monofocal IOL calculated for distance. Unfortunately, this may not be acceptable for most patients because their original journey was a trip to spectacle

Henderson BA, Yoo SH. *Curbside Consultation in Refractive and Lens-Based Surgery: 49 Clinical Questions* (pp 199-200)
© 2015 SLACK Incorporated

independence land and this option implies a generalized failure of the procedure. Other options includes a version of monovision with either implantation of a standard monofocal IOL aiming for –1.50 to –2.00 or implantation of an accommodative IOL aiming for –0.75 to –1.50, depending on the level of near acuity achieved with the first eye.

Before proceeding with monovision surgically, it would be nice to demonstrate monovision to patients with a contact lens trial; this will depend on their level of preoperative visual acuity. As part of the preoperative informed consent, a thorough discussion of the limitations of all IOL options, including the possibility and expense of corneal refractive enhancements, second eye monovision, and mixing and matching various presbyopia IOL models should be reviewed. I believe that for most patients who are willing to pay the expense of an accommodative IOL in the second eye, the accommodative IOL offers the best option over a standard monofocal IOL because less postoperative myopia can be targeted, and up to 1 diopter (D) of possible accommodative effect may still be achieved in the second eye.

The final option for this patient with unacceptable near acuity in his or her first eye would be implantation of a multifocal IOL in the second eye.[2] This is a more drastic and possibly problematic option because the patient may become unhappy with the first eye due to limited near vision and unhappy with the second eye due to the optical aberrations of multifocality—a nightmarish double whammy of dissatisfaction. Before proceeding down this road, the surgeon needs to again have an indepth discussion with the patient and get a good feeling about how this particular patient might respond to the optical shortcomings and adaptation of mixing and matching a monofocal accommodative IOL with a multifocal IOL. A patient who is not fully aware of the reasons for limited near vision in the first eye or is irate due to the result in the first eye should not have a multifocal IOL in the second eye. In my clinic, patients who receive an accommodative IOL in their first eye usually had a good reason for receiving this model over a multifocal IOL, including ocular pathology, unreasonable expectations, or an inability to have an intelligent informed discussion regarding the limitations and aberrations inherent in multifocal technology. These patients obviously should not have a multifocal IOL implanted in their second eye and would be best served with an accommodative IOL aiming for partial monovision.

With our current options for presbyopia-correcting IOLs, choosing the right lens for the right patient is still more art than science. Selecting cooperative, highly motivated patients goes a long way to reduce both patient and surgeon stress, especially when the desired outcome is not achieved. An honest preoperative discussion of the limitations of the various IOLs, in addition to reviewing the options for altering the surgical plan in the second eye, will ultimately yield a higher percentage of patients who are content with their final results.

References

1. Mesci C, Erbil HH, Olgun A, Yaylali SA. Visual performances with monofocal, accommodating, and multifocal intraocular lenses in patients with unilateral cataract. *Am J Ophthalmol*. 2010;150:609-618.
2. Pepose JS, Qazi MA, Davies J, et al. Visual performance of patients with bilateral vs combination Crystalens, ReZoom, and ReSTOR intraocular lens implants. *Am J Ophthalmol*. 2007;144:347-357.

FINANCIAL DISCLOSURES

Dr. *Alessandro Abbouda* has no financial or proprietary interest in the materials presented herein.

Dr. *Natalie Afshari* has not disclosed any relevant financial relationships.

Dr. *Jorge L. Alió* has no financial or proprietary interest in the materials presented herein.

Dr. *Zaina Al-Mohtaseb* has no financial or proprietary interest in the materials presented herein.

Dr. *Renato Ambrósio Jr* is a consultant to Oculus.

Dr. *Samuel Arba Mosquera* is an employee for SCHWIND eye-tech-solutions, manufacturer of the AMARIS system.

Dr. *John P. Berdahl* has no financial or proprietary interest in the materials presented herein.

Dr. *Hiroko Bissen-Miyajima* has no financial or proprietary interest in the materials presented herein.

Dr. *Ofelia Brugnoli de Pagano* has no financial or proprietary interest in the materials presented herein.

Dr. *Florence Cabot* has no financial or proprietary interest in the materials presented herein.

Dr. *Francesco Carones* has no financial or proprietary interest in the materials presented herein.

Dr. *Jessica B. Ciralsky* is a consultant for Alcon, Allergan, and Abbott Medical Optics.

Dr. *Rosane de Oliveira Corrêa* has no financial or proprietary interest in the materials presented herein.

Dr. *William W. Culbertson* has no financial or proprietary interest in the materials presented herein.

Dr. Yassine J. Daoud has no financial or proprietary interest in the materials presented herein.

Dr. Mahshad Darvish-Zargar has no financial or proprietary interest in the materials presented herein.

Dr. Elizabeth A. Davis is a consultant for Abbott Medical Optics, a speaker for Bausch + Lomb, and holds stock in Refractec.

Dr. Uday Devgan has no financial or proprietary interest in the materials presented herein.

Dr. Deepinder K. Dhaliwal has no financial or proprietary interest in the materials presented herein.

Dr. Vasilios F. Diakonis has no financial or proprietary interest in the materials presented herein.

Dr. Eric D. Donnenfeld is a consultant for Allergan, Bausch + Lomb, Tearlab, and RPS.

Dr. Jason N. Edmonds has no financial or proprietary interest in the materials presented herein.

Dr. Damien Gatinel has not disclosed any relevant financial relationships.

Dr. Ramon Coral Ghanem has no financial or proprietary interest in the materials presented herein.

Dr. Vinícius Coral Ghanem has no financial or proprietary interest in the materials presented herein.

Dr. Preeya K. Gupta has no financial or proprietary interest in the materials presented herein.

Dr. David R. Hardten has no financial or proprietary interest in the materials presented herein.

Dr. Lingmin He has served as a consultant for Auris Surgical Robotics and Oculeve, Inc.

Dr. Bonnie An Henderson is a consultant for Alcon, Bausch + Lomb, Abbott Medical Optics, and Genzyme.

Dr. Richard S. Hoffman has no financial or proprietary interest in the materials presented herein.

Dr. Edward J. Holland is a consultant for Abbott Medical Optics, Alcon Laboratories, Inc., Bausch + Lomb, Senju Pharmaceutical Co., LTD., Wavetec Vision Systems, Inc., SARCode, and TearScience; he has received lecture fees from Alcon Laboratories, Inc. and Bausch + Lomb; he has received grant support from Abbott Medical Optics, Alcon Laboratories, Inc., and Wavetec Vision Systems, Inc.

Dr. Yoshihiko Iida has no financial or proprietary interest in the materials presented herein.

Dr. A.J. Kanellopoulos is a consultant for Alcon, Avedro, Allergan, and I-Optics.

Dr. Vardhaman P. Kankariya has no financial or proprietary interest in the materials presented herein.

Dr. Sumitra S. Khandelwal has no financial or proprietary interest in the materials presented herein.

Dr. Wei Boon Khor has no financial or proprietary interest in the materials presented herein.

Dr. Jae Yong Kim has no financial or proprietary interest in the materials presented herein.

Dr. Terry Kim has no financial or proprietary interest in the materials presented herein.

Dr. Michael C. Knorz has no financial or proprietary interest in the materials presented herein.

Dr. Douglas D. Koch has not disclosed any relevant financial relationships.

Dr. George A. Kontadakis has no financial or proprietary interest in the materials presented herein.

Dr. George D. Kymionis has no financial or proprietary interest in the materials presented herein.

Dr. Edward C. Lai is a consultant for Allergan.

Dr. Richard L. Lindstrom is a consultant for Alcon, Abbott Medical Optics, and Bausch + Lomb.

Dr. Jordon G. Lubahn has no financial or proprietary interest in the materials presented herein.

Dr. Kim-Binh Mai has no financial or proprietary interest in the materials presented herein.

Dr. Alex Mammen has no financial or proprietary interest in the materials presented herein.

Dr. Edward E. Manche a consultant for Gerson Lehrmann, Oculeve, Inc., and Best Doctors, Inc. and am an equity owner in Calhoun Vision, Inc., Veralas, Inc., Seros Medical, LLC., Krypton Vision, Inc. and Refresh Innovations, Inc.

Dr. Jay J. Meyer has no financial or proprietary interest in the materials presented herein.

Dr. Kevin M. Miller is a consultant and clinical investigator for Alcon Laboratories, which makes the Verion system. Dr. Miller also helped Epsilon develop the ET-04 toric marker and has his name on it, but receives no royalties or income from its sale.

Dr. Majid Moshirfar has no financial or proprietary interest in the materials presented herein.

Dr. Afshan Nanji has no financial or proprietary interest in the materials presented herein.

Dr. Louis D. "Skip" Nichamin has no financial or proprietary interest in the materials presented herein.

Dr. Rudy M. M. A. Nuijts is a consultant for Alcon, TheaPharma and ASICO; he has received study grants from Acufocus, Alcon, Carl Zeiss, Ophtec and Physiol; and received a lecture fee from Alcon.

Dr. Mark Packer is a consultant for Advanced Vision Science, Inc., Aerie Pharmaceuticals, Inc., Allergan, Inc., Bausch + Lomb (Valeant Pharmaceuticals International, Inc.), Lensar, Inc., PowerVision, Inc., Oculeve, Inc., Rayner Intraocular Lenses, Ltd., Refocus Group, Inc., Reichert, Inc., STAAR Surgical Company, Inc., Transcend Medical, Inc., TrueVision Systems, Inc., VisionCare Ophthalmic Technologies, Inc., and WaveTec Vision Systems, Inc. Dr. Packer has equity in Angle, LLC, Corinthian Ophthalmic, Inc., Iantech, Inc., Lensar, Inc., mTuitive, Inc., Surgiview, LLC, Transcend Medical, Inc., TrueVision Systems, Inc., WaveTec Vision Systems, Inc.

Dr. Gabriela L. Pagano has no financial or proprietary interest in the materials presented herein.

Dr. Parag Parekh has no financial or proprietary interest in the materials presented herein.

Dr. Jay S. Pepose is consultant for Abbott Medical Optics, Alcon, and Bausch + Lomb.

Dr. J. Bradley Randleman has no financial or proprietary interest in the materials presented herein.

Dr. Peter A. Rapoza has no financial or proprietary interest in the materials presented herein.

Dr. Sherman Reeves is a consultant for Abbott Medical Optics and Allergan.

Dr. Alain Saad has no financial or proprietary interest in the materials presented herein.

Dr. Matthew J. Schear has no financial or proprietary interest in the materials presented herein.

Dr. Kimiya Shimizu has no financial or proprietary interest in the materials presented herein.

Dr. Walter J. Stark has no financial or proprietary interest in the materials presented herein.

Dr. Roger F. Steinert is a consultant to Abbott Medical Optics.

Dr. Richard Tipperman is a consultant to Alcon Laboratories.

Dr. William Trattler is a consultant to Oculus.

Dr. Pravin Krishna Vaddavalli has no financial or proprietary interest in the materials presented herein.

Dr. Bruna V. Ventura has no financial or proprietary interest in the materials presented herein.

Dr. Laura Vickers has no financial or proprietary interest in the materials presented herein.

Dr. Nienke Visser has no financial or proprietary interest in the materials presented herein.

Dr. R. Bruce Wallace III has not disclosed any relevant financial relationships.

Dr. Li Wang has no financial or proprietary interest in the materials presented herein.

Dr. Matthew J. Weiss has no financial or proprietary interest in the materials presented herein.

Dr. Sonia H. Yoo is a consultant for Alcon, Abbott Medical Optics, Bausch + Lomb, Allergan, Carl Zeiss Meditec and Transcend Medical

Dr. Roberto Zaldivar has no financial or proprietary interest in the materials presented herein.

Dr. Roger Zaldivar has no financial or proprietary interest in the materials presented herein.

INDEX